As an ENT (ear, nose, and throat) physician, I found *Sinus Survival* to be both accurate and informative. There is no other book that I am aware of which is as thorough and helpful in educating people about their sinuses. I will gladly recommend it to my patients.

J. Birney, M.D.—Littleton, CO

A primary responsibility of a family physician is patient education. *Sinus Survival* helps people to quickly recognize a sinus infection, to treat their own sinus condition, and to practice preventive medicine on their sinuses. This book is not only a gift for patients, but will make my job much easier as well.

H. Brodie, M.D.—Littleton, CO

What a treat to read your book, *Sinus Survival*. I have had chronic sinusitis for 46 years. I have gotten used to the situation and have more or less learned to live with it. Thank you for a wonderful approach to sinus care for the professional as well as the lay person.

T. Jerman, R.N.—Lakewood, CO

I am really excited about *Sinus Survival*. As a pharmacist, I am asked questions on a daily basis about sinuses. Your book has helped me tremendously, and I can now pass that information on to my customers. I'd like to have the book for sale in my pharmacy as well.

T. Caruso, R.Ph.—Monument, CO

SINUS SURVIVAL

A Complete Guide to Caring for America's Most Common Ailment

Revised Edition

Dr. Robert S. Ivker

WHOLE HEALTH PRESS
Littleton, Colorado

Published 1988. Revised Edition 1991.

Printed in the United States of America on recycled paper.
ISBN 0-9621845-1-9

Illustrations by Eileen Rudnick

Cover photograph: A winter day in Denver, Colorado. Air quality on this day was rated "acceptable."
Photo by Robert S. Ivker

To my father, Morris,
whose love of medicine has been
an inspiration to me, and whose lifelong chronic
sinusitis he so generously shared with me.

THANKS TO:

Ross Barrick and Richard Crowther for educating me about the risks of and remedies for indoor air pollution.

Zach Brinkerhoff for the introduction to reflexology.

Deepak Chopra, Brugh Joy, Elisabeth Kubler-Ross, Evarts Loomis, Emmett Miller, Dean Ornish, Norm Shealy, and Bernie Siegel for their courage in blazing the trail for holistic medicine.

Paul Feldman for pushing hard enough to get me started on this project.

Wilbur Flachman, Bonnie Meadows, Annette Allen, and the rest of the staff of The Publishing House for their guidance in creating the book from a manuscript.

Carl Flaxer, my real-life Marcus Welby, M.D.

Sylvia Flesner for expanding my vision and providing several of the tools with which I healed my sinuses.

Ken Gerdes for his enthusiasm and support, and for his wisdom in recognizing the link between the environment and chronic disease.

Morty Goldman for sharing his dream and helping me to discover the meaning of fun. I will e'er remember.

Patty Hodgins for her superb job of editing both editions.

Milton Ivker and Janice Birney for their technical input and for reassuring me that *Sinus Survival* made good sense to otolaryngologists.

George Kitchie, Kathy Fisher, and Bonnie Katz for teaching me about Chinese medicine.

Apisai Lailai for demonstrating so powerfully what holistic health looks and feels like.

Myron McClellan for helping me to realize that anything is possible, even curing chronic sinusitis.

Joel Miller and Joe Stapen for giving me greater clarity on the meaning of mental and emotional health.

Susan and Steve Morris, Charlie Cropley, and Todd Nelson for sharing their knowledge of naturopathic and homeopathic medicine.

Doug Shapiro for lending his body, and especially his sinuses, to science.

Bill Silvers for his editing, encouragement, and expertise on noses, sinuses, allergies, and asthma.

Luana Veo, Jaison Kayn, and Jeff Durland for providing me with the opportunity to experience the healing potential of breath therapy and bodywork.

The many patients who taught me most of what I know about sinus disease.

The women in my life—Thelma, for being such an outstanding teacher of caring and parenting; and Harriet, Julie, and Carin, whose love, understanding, and support have helped make this book a reality.

God for bringing all of these people into my life.

Table of Contents

Introduction

Sinus disease is a problem not easily recognized by either doctor or patient. Most people with a sinus infection believe they have "a cold that just won't quit." In this book I offer a clinical diagnosis for both acute and chronic sinusitis.

In my medical career I have been responsible for the care of more than 20,000 patients with sinus disease. From 1977 to 1987, I worked hard on my own sinus condition (more about that later) and with my patients to dispel the belief that I and they would have to live indefinitely with the unpleasantness of the condition—despite the fact that conventional methods of treating it were becoming increasingly less effective.

Throughout the ten-year treatment program I used for my own sinus disease, I experimented with a myriad of therapeutic modalities, innovative techniques, and folk remedies. The bulk of my work was based upon medical science, and those methods that were effective are all contained in this book. This approach vastly improved my sinuses; however, it was not until my healing journey took me into the exciting new frontier of holistic medicine that I obtained a cure. I have not had a sinus infection nor any of the symptoms of chronic sinusitis for almost four years. Since publishing the original edition of *Sinus Survival,* I have had the opportunity to treat some of the most challenging sinus patients I've ever seen. They too are experiencing remarkable results. Through working with them, I have been able to refine some of the material from that first edition.

The need to practice "sinus survival" began for me in 1975 with my first sinus infection. I had suffered with seasonal allergies (hay fever) throughout most of my childhood, but this was something very different. Over the next three years, I had several more infections and developed chronic sinusitis as well. "Normal" for me now meant a stuffy head, frequent sinus headaches, and lots of mucus drainage down the back of my throat. I consulted an ear, nose, and throat (ENT) specialist who basically told me that there was no cure and that I would "have to learn to live with it." I was stunned.

As a young physician who staunchly believed in the healing power of medical science, I had gotten a strong dose of reality. Although I had hardly been given a death sentence, sinus disease was having a profound impact on the quality of my life. The specialist's statement was a rude reminder that, although modern medicine is saving many lives and performing "miracles" daily, we are only able to cure about 25 percent of the ailments treated. Chronic sinusitis is not among that select group.

Ironically, it was to enhance the quality of my life that I came to Denver, Colorado, in 1972. There I entered a family practice residency training program, where I was taught that as a family doctor, it was part of my responsibility to teach my patients about health and preventive medicine—how to stay well.

During my three years at Mercy Medical Center, I felt exhilarated whenever I caught a glimpse of the magnificent Rocky Mountains on the western edge of the city. I also distinctly recall my disappointment and disgust when, with increasing frequency, that vista was obstructed with what later came to be known as the brown cloud. Air pollution was becoming a problem that Denver could no longer ignore.

After completing the residency, I took my family and newly developed sinus condition to the outskirts of the city, where I began a solo family practice. Being something of a statistician, I kept track of the diagnoses of all of my patients. Through the mid- to late 1970s, acute sinusitis (sinus infection) was usually fourteenth or fifteenth on my list of the top twenty diagnoses. By 1982 it had become number one, and it has headed the list ever since. In compiling data from other family practices and residencies throughout the country for a medical conference I was organizing, I found that my observation correlated with those of other family doctors. Sinusitis was near the top of every list of the most common ailments being treated by family physicians. In the summer of 1981, the National Center for Health Statistics reported that for the first time in its statistic-taking history, chronic sinusitis had become the most common chronic disease in the United States, more common than arthritis. Today nearly *one out of every seven Americans* (33.7 million people) is a sinus sufferer. Sinus disease has become an epidemic right under (and around) our noses.

I asked myself, "Why this sudden epidemic of sinus disease?" The answer came from above—it was the toxic cloud hovering over the city like a suffocating blanket and invading homes and workplaces to create increasingly polluted indoor air. There was no escape. Of course, residents of the Mile High City are not alone in their suffering: Almost every major urban center in the world is plagued with air pollution.

In the United States alone, the Environmental Protection Agency (EPA) has reported, more than 150 million Americans (60 percent of the U.S. population) live in areas where the air is hazardous to their health. But what is actually happening to us as a result of breathing this filthy air? That question has still not been addressed by any governmental agency. Part of my purpose in writing this book has been to offer my own theory about the devastating impact air pollution is having on human beings. In this revised edition I have included a section on indoor air pollution, a subject the EPA is now addressing as it identifies the multitude of air pollutants found in our homes and workplaces.

Although it has not yet been conclusively proven in a laboratory, the air pollution–sinus disease connection will certainly withstand any scientific scrutiny. A primary function of the sinuses in their job of protecting our lungs is to filter the air we breathe. We need only look at what we're breathing to appreciate that our sinuses are, at the very least, having to work much harder than they used to. After I first published this book late in 1988, I was invited to speak to the scientists at the Air Pollution Health Effects Laboratory at the University of California-Irvine. The director of the lab, Dr. Robert F. Phalen, reported to me, "There is scientific evidence relating air pollution to significant epithelial cell damage in the nasal cavity of the rat." This is solid scientific support for the pollution–sinus disease link.

Sales of this book in bookstores and in physicians' (ENT

specialists and family practitioners) offices have shown an interesting pattern. Sales have been highest in the cities and states that the EPA has identified as having the dirtiest air—Los Angeles, Denver, Ohio, Texas, Michigan, Illinois, Tennessee, and Indiana. This sales pattern may not be too scientific, but it will surely score some circumstantial points in support of my theory.

Using this book, readers will be able to diagnose, treat, prevent, and—if they choose to make that level of commitment—cure themselves of the affliction of sinus disease. It is a condition that easily lends itself to self-healing. Those readers who do not have a sinus problem will learn of the potential hazards of breathing polluted air and what they can do to protect themselves from it through the practice of preventive medicine. *Sinus Survival* provides a practical plan for living a full and healthy lifestyle in an increasingly unhealthy environment.

This book offers you many avenues of possible relief from sinus disease. They all work. In Part I you may choose from a multitude of options that offer rapid improvement of symptoms. Part II deals more with the treatment of causes and allows you to take increased responsibility not only for the condition of your sinuses but also for your overall state of health. The methods described take a bit longer to implement and require more effort, but the depth of improvement in your sinuses and health in general will be far greater. Start with Part I and if you are happy with the results, then move on to Part II. The holistic program is a personalized approach to health. It is based upon learning to love yourself in all of the components of your life—physical, mental, emotional, spiritual, and social. Loving yourself is not a selfish indulgence, but rather a means of discovering, appreciating, and accepting the unique individual that you are. Through this work you will be able to better learn what feels good to you, how to provide it for yourself and how to give more to others. You will begin to experience a greater degree of health and vitality than you've ever had before.

Part I

The Basics of Sinus Disease

Chapter 1

What Are Sinuses?

Most people probably assume that the word "sinus" means "nose." They would be close, both anatomically and physiologically; but although the nose and sinuses are connected, they are separate parts of the body. The sinuses are air-filled cavities located behind and around the nose and eyes. They are medically referred to as the air sinuses or paranasal sinuses. There are usually four sets, roughly divided in half for each side of the head. The halves may be asymmetrical in size and shape.

The sinuses are identified as frontal, maxillary, sphenoid, and ethmoid (Figure A). The frontal sinuses lie above the eyes just above the nose and behind the forehead. The maxillaries, the largest of the sinuses, are pyramid-shaped cavities located inside each cheekbone. The ethmoids are multicompartmental sinuses behind the maxillaries and between the bony orbits of the eyes. They are complex labyrinths of small air pockets. The sphenoids are situated deep in the skull behind the nose, slightly below the ethmoids. The ethmoidal, sphenoidal, and maxillary sinuses are all present at birth, although the latter do not reach full development until a person is sixteen to twenty-one years of age. The frontal sinuses are not present until the age of eight.

To make mucus drainage and air exchange possible, each sinus is connected to the nasal passage by a thin duct about the size of a pencil lead. The ducts of the maxillaries are located at the top of the sinus, making drainage difficult and blockage easy. A series of small ducts in the nasal wall drain the ethmoid sinuses, and these openings are also easily blocked. The openings of the ducts are called ostia, and they average about two millimeters in diameter. Although most of the human body seems to have been created perfectly, the maxillary sinuses are a distinct exception. They appear to be better suited to four-legged animals, particularly with regard to the position of the

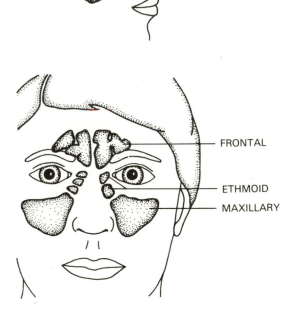

Figure A. Location of Sinuses.

ostia. As upright posture evolved, ease of sinus drainage diminished.

The same kind of tissue, called respiratory epithelium, lines all of the sinuses, the nose, and the lungs. In fact, these three are all part of the respiratory tract (Figure B), that system of the body involved with the essential function of breathing. The outermost part of the epithelium is called the mucosa; this is a continuous mucous-membrane lining the sinuses, ducts, and nasal passages. Therefore, anything that causes a swelling in

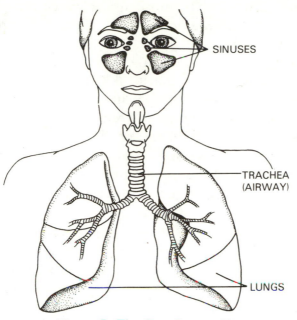

Figure B. The Respiratory Tract.

the nose can similarly affect the sinuses. On the surface of this membrane are cilia (microscopic hairlike filaments) that maintain a constant sweeping motion to remove the watery discharge called mucus (Figure C).

The mucous membrane and its cilia provide a good defensive mechanism against infections. The entire mucus covering of the maxillary sinus is normally cleared every ten minutes. The membrane produces between a pint and a quart of mucus daily. The mucus traps particles entering the nasal passage for the cilia to sweep toward the back of the nose, where the particles are swallowed and destroyed by stomach acids.

No one within the medical community seems able to scientifically state the exact function of the sinuses. (There is agreement, however, that they lighten the weight of the skull.) By virtue of their location and structure (anatomy) and the micro-anatomy and function of the mucous membrane, most physicians would agree with the following conclusions. All these conclusions have frequently been alluded to in the medical literature, although never proven in a laboratory.

The sinuses, along with the nose, as the upper part of the respiratory tract, *serve as the body's chief protector of the lungs.* They do this by acting as a *"filter"*—helping to defend against viruses, dirt and dust particles, allergens, and anything else in the air that would be harmful to the lungs; as a *"humidifier"*—by moistening dry air that would be irritating to the lungs; and as a *"temperature regulator"*—by cooling excessively hot air and warming extremely cold air that would be a shock to the lungs. We inhale about 17,000 times a day, moving about two gallons of air per minute. The nose and sinuses are very busy protectors and are always at work shielding the lungs from harm. Our lungs are the primary vehicle through which our bodies obtain oxygen—the most vital element in maintaining good health and life itself.

The sinuses, as the body's leading defenders against injury and/or illness to the lungs, have been neglected both by the medical community and by its patients. Think about a quarterback on the football field whose offensive line is weak and beginning to break down. He may not be killed, literally, but what about his health and the quality of his life? Our sinuses are being assaulted and are beginning to deteriorate. The health of our lungs, and ultimately our bodies, is at stake. Let us see how we might help preserve good health by reinforcing our first line of defense, the sinuses.

Chapter 2

What Makes Sinuses Sick?

The factors that will be discussed in this chapter have the potential to adversely affect any sinus. However, the person who has had previous sinus problems or who has weakened sinuses for any of the reasons mentioned in this chapter is at highest risk for developing sinusitis. The following factors are involved: the common cold, cigarettes and other sources of smoke, air pollution, dry air, cold air, fumes, allergies, occupational hazards, dental problems, immunodeficiency, malformations, and emotional stress.

THE COMMON COLD

The story of what often becomes a lifetime of "sinus problems" usually begins with the common cold. Normally, air and mucus flow freely along the ducts connecting the nose and sinuses. Trouble starts when the system becomes obstructed, usually by a cold. This obstruction occurs as a result of inflammation and swelling of the nasal mucous membrane. The cold virus inactivates the cilia of the nasal membrane, causing the mucus in the nose to stagnate rather than flow (Figure C). As a result, the mucus being produced in the sinuses cannot drain properly, and the sinuses become a breeding ground for bacteria. This pooling of stagnant mucus can easily result in a sinus infection, especially in individuals who have had such infections previously.

Through the early and mid-1970s, I treated many patients who had nothing more than a "bad cold." However, by the late seventies and especially early eighties, patients with the common cold became less frequent visitors to my office. They were being replaced by patients who greeted me with com-

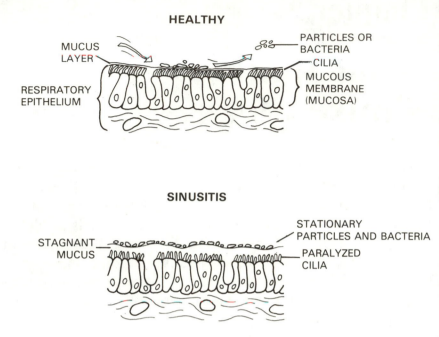

Figure C. The Sinus Lining.

plaints like, "Doctor, I have had this cold for the past two weeks now" (or three weeks or several months, or in a few cases, a year or more!). These people usually had sinusitis, and not until they had completed a course of antibiotics were they able to rid themselves of their "cold." It also became quite apparent that subsequent to their first infection, those who had never before had a sinus infection were now frequently returning with the same problem. As a result of that first bout with sinusitis, the mucous membrane and especially the cilia are left in a somewhat damaged and weakened state. For many, the membrane never completely recovers, especially in an environment that is harsh on the sinuses. What I have been observing with increasing frequency is that one or two "bad colds" can potentially result in a permanently weak sinus, i.e., chronic sinusitis. This impaired sinus then becomes much more susceptible to additional infections, as a result of a cold or any of the other risk factors that I will now describe.

CIGARETTES AND OTHER SOURCES OF SMOKE

Whenever a patient with a sinus infection returns to my office two or more weeks after completing a course of anti-biotics and complains to me, "Doctor, I'm not any better," my first response is always the question, "Have you been smoking?" Often, the patient answers yes. It is extremely difficult to have healthy sinuses if you smoke cigarettes. Nicotine paralyzes the cilia. I would be hard pressed to name anything more harmful to the body's air filter than smoke of any kind that is inhaled or exhaled through the nose. Cigarette smoke is most often involved, but cigar, pipe, campfire, and cooking smoke are also frequent villains. Marijuana and especially cocaine (both smoked and snorted) are also quite harmful to the nasal mucous membrane.

If you are curious what smoke does to the sinuses, take a look at a used cigarette filter. It will give you some idea of what is happening not only to the sinuses, but to the lungs as well. What is occurring at the tissue level is that the smoke causes irritation of the mucous membrane. The weaker the sinus (i.e., usually one that has been infected previously), the greater the level of irritation. The greater the irritation, the more inflamed the mucous membrane becomes. Inflammation of the mucous membrane results in its swelling, increased mucus secretion, and damage to the cilia. This swelling can potentially cause obstruction of the sinuses, which then produces a condition in the sinuses very similar to that created by the common cold (Figure C).

The principle described here of body fluids being obstructed holds true for almost any part of the human body. Whether it is the bladder, bowel, lung, kidney, or middle ear space, when fluids or secretions are unable to drain normally, the potential for infection is high. This likely scenario of infection in the sinuses can be triggered not only by the common cold and cigarette smoke, but almost all of the other factors that I will mention later in this chapter. This is a theory that the medical establishment has not yet proven. It is presently beyond the scope of science to microscopically observe what is happening to the mucous membrane in someone's sinus as it is being suffocated with smoke. However, as with the speculation on the function of the sinuses, this theory, too, would have strong support among most physicians.

For those of you who are sinus sufferers and do not smoke, and therefore may not have been paying close attention, I am sorry to say that even you are not immune to the problems generated by smoke. Studies in recent years have shown that non-smokers who live or work with smokers are adversely affected. New laws that prohibit cigarette smoking in public places are helping, but we have a long way to go in this endeavor.

AIR POLLUTION—OUTDOOR

I was struck by a comment made by one of the Apollo astronauts several years ago following his mission. He said that the most disturbing part of his flight was seeing a grayish haze over almost every land mass on earth. What was this mysterious ugly blanket covering our beautiful planet? No explanation was given. One could only guess at the answer.

However, living in Denver gave me a good clue. The "Mile-High City," one of this country's most polluted metropolitan areas, is often covered by a thick brownish-gray pall of smog known locally as the brown cloud. Most cities in the world are similarly afflicted with significant air pollution. In mountainous areas where temperature inversions are frequent; in cities where diesel fuel is used extensively, especially in Europe; in the heavily industrialized northeast corridor of the United States; and in most areas where there are coal-fired power plants, the problem of air pollution is even more acute. Almost every country in the world is now familiar with this rapidly growing dilemma. Is it possible that it has reached such immense proportions that it is visible from space? Even more important, what is this filthy air doing to the human beings who have created the problem?

Since the early 1970s, the incidence of acute sinusitis has risen dramatically in Denver. In my practice, it has consistently been the most common ailment since 1982. Is it only a coincidence that air pollution has undergone a similar meteoric rise during the same period of time? The pollution is most acute from mid-November to mid-January, when temperature inversions (warm air aloft trapping cold air and pollutants near the ground) are most common. This also happens to be the time of year when we see the greatest number of sinus infections. Many people who work in center city or in other high-pollution areas are aware of the connection between their sinus congestion and sinus headaches on particularly bad pollution days.

There is scientific evidence to implicate carbon monoxide as the most dangerous element of air pollution. Why? Because in high enough concentrations, it is capable of killing people with weak hearts and lungs. It is also the most often measured component of air pollution, and about 25 percent of it comes from vehicle emissions. But carbon monoxide is an odorless and colorless gas. What is that stuff that we can see—the brown cloud—and what is it doing to the sinuses of us healthy people when we breathe it?

Visible pollution consists primarily of the following elements: particulates, oxides of sulfur, oxides of nitrogen, hydrocarbons, and ozone. Particulates are tiny particles of solid and liquid material—dust, sand, cinders, soot, smoke, and liquid droplets—found in the atmosphere. They come from a variety of sources, including roads, farm fields, construction sites, factories, power plants, fireplaces, wood-burning stoves, windblown dust, and diesel and car exhaust. When inhaled, larger particles (greater than ten microns in diameter) are known to lodge in the nose and sinuses. After all, what is a filter for? Oxides of sulfur, especially sulfur dioxide (a colorless gas with a rotten-egg odor), are typically transformed into particulates. They are emitted mainly by coal- and oil-fired power plants, refineries, pulp and paper mills, and nonferrous smelters. They are a major contributor to acid rain. Sulfur oxides are finer particles (less than ten microns in diameter—see Figure E in Chapter 8) and are also the responsibility of the filtering sinuses. Unfortunately, there is a price to be paid for protecting the lungs from this toxic substance. Sulfur oxide particles can easily penetrate the mucosal lining, and studies have shown that they have an intensely irritating effect on the bronchial mucosa (whose tissue is the same type as the sinuses), resulting in damage to the cilia and initiation of bronchitis. If sulfur oxides can cause bronchitis in the lungs, would an assumption that they can also cause sinusitis be too far-fetched?

According to the 1988 National Air Quality and Emissions Trends Report, published by the EPA, the metropolitan areas with the highest average particulate concentrations that year were (in descending order) Riverside–San Bernardino, California; St. Louis, Missouri; Tucson, Arizona; Los Angeles–Long Beach, California and Las Vegas, Nevada. Those with the highest amounts of sulfur dioxide were Steubenville, Ohio–Weirton, West Virginia; Pittsburgh, Pennsylvania; New York City; Salt Lake City, Utah; and Evansville, Indiana.

Nitrogen oxides are the primary components of photochemical smog. Their principal constituent is nitrogen dioxide, a yellowish-brown, highly reactive gas. Nitrogen oxides form when fuel is burned at high temperatures—when combustion occurs. The two major emissions sources are internal combustion engines—motor vehicles and aircraft—and stationary fuel combustion sources such as electric utilities and industrial boilers. Like sulfur oxides, nitrogen oxides can irritate the lungs, causing ciliary paralysis, bronchitis, and pneumonia. They are also capable of impairing the body's immune defenses against bacterial and viral infection.

Los Angeles County is the only area in the country exceeding the federal nitrogen dioxide standard. The other cities that are highest in this pollutant are Riverside–San Bernardino, California; Anaheim, California; Denver, Colorado; Philadelphia, Pennsylvania; and Memphis, Tennessee.

Hydrocarbons are evaporated or incompletely burned organic compounds. The largest sources of hydrocarbons in the atmosphere include internal combustion engines, certain industrial processes (such as coke ovens in steel mills), and evaporation of liquids (such as gasoline in fuel transfers, and industrial and household solvents). Hydrocarbons are known to be highly irritating to the mucous membrane.

Ozone is the major component of smog. It is produced when sunlight acts upon nitrogen oxides and hydrocarbons. The many sources of both these substances have already been mentioned. Ozone in the lower, breathable part of the atmosphere (within 1000 feet of the earth's surface) is harmful to human and animal health, crops, and forests. In the upper atmosphere, ozone is beneficial, absorbing the harmful rays (ultraviolet-B) of sunlight. The continuing depletion of the upper ozone layer has become a serious health concern. Unfortunately, harmful ozone in the lower air does not move up to replenish the deteriorating ozone layer in the higher reaches of our atmosphere.

Ozone in the lower atmosphere is one of our most serious environmental challenges. Few, if any, urban areas are free of it. Four broad geographic regions are seriously affected: southern California (by far the worst), the Northeast (especially the New York City area), the Texas Gulf Coast, and the Chicago-Milwaukee area. The top five cities are Los Angeles-Long Beach, Riverside-San Bernardino, Anaheim-Santa Ana, Houston, and Bridgeport-Milford, Connecticut.

A growing body of scientific data indicates that ozone is a significant risk to human health. It has been shown to affect not only people with impaired respiratory systems, such as asthmatics, but also many people with healthy lungs, both children and adults. It can cause shortness of breath and coughing when healthy adults are exercising and more serious effects in the young, old, and infirm. Almost all of the scientific research has been done on lungs. But at the Air Pollution Health Effects Laboratory at the University of California-Irvine, nasal effects have also been studied. To my knowledge there has not been any direct research on the sinuses. However, from the findings at this laboratory on the nasal cavities of rats, there is substantial support for the connection between air pollution (at least ozone) and sinus disease. The laboratory has found significant damage to the mucous membrane surrounding the opening to the maxillary sinuses as a result of inhaling ozone. This could easily lead to the obstruction of the sinuses and subsequent infection.

Nowhere in the United States is the problem of air pollution more acute than in Los Angeles. (Not coincidentally, sales of *Sinus Survival* have been greater in that area than anywhere else.) A recent study on ten- and eleven-year-olds in Los Angeles revealed that their lung capacity is already diminished by 17 percent compared to the normal range for that age. A pathologist at the University of Southern California, in performing autopsies on Los Angeles children killed accidentally, is finding a disturbing frequency of emphysematous changes previously seen only in adult lungs. But Los Angeles is not unique. Other areas of the country are well on their way to matching that city's severity of pollution and its damaging effect on the lungs.

Conspicuous by its absence in the medical and scientific literature is any mention of the chief protector of the lungs—the sinuses. How much evidence is necessary before we begin to recognize the magnitude of this problem? We are being given ample warning. The chief defender of our lungs is breaking down in epidemic numbers. There is already a dramatic increase in the incidence of lung disease—asthma, emphysema, and lung cancer. Most physicians rate air pollution second only to cigarettes as a cause of this trend. Americans are certainly not alone in suffering with this plague of pollution. According to the World Health Organization, cities such as New Delhi, India; Seoul, Korea; and Mexico City are far worse than Los Angeles. Dying forests across central Europe are a testament to the air pollution of that heavily industrialized continent. Huge demonstrations demanding a cleanup of air pollution have been reported in many Soviet cities.

But no one else can do it for us. Of course there are solutions: Most entail changing our lifestyle. In 1950, there were 50 million cars worldwide, 75 percent of them in the United States. This number doubled by 1960, redoubled by 1970, and doubled again by 1990—an eightfold increase, to 400 million cars. U.S. drivers now own only one-third of the world's total, but one-half of all Americans have put two cars in their garage. We have created a monster and it is literally killing us and the planet we live on. Automobiles, along with trucks and buses, are the chief source of our air pollution. The availability and use of alternative fuels—ethanol, methanol, hydrogen, and natural gas—would make a profound difference. Greater enforcement of engine emission tests, development of mass transit sytems, participation in carpooling, and construction of bicycle paths, along with the conversion of power plants from coal to natural gas, the development of solar energy, and a mass reduction of wood burning, are all measures that would have an immediate impact on cleaning our air.

There is nothing more critical to human survival than the quality of the air we breathe. Many of us are already suffering the ill effects of breathing unhealthy air. If each of us can do at least one thing to decrease air pollution, then collectively we can cure this disease.

AIR POLLUTION—INDOOR

Unfortunately, no one can escape from the plague of dirty air by remaining indoors. The EPA has identified a multitude of indoor air pollutants, not the least of which is outdoor air—our primary source of indoor ventilation air. Subsequent to a study concluded in November 1988, the EPA reported that indoor air can be as much as 100 times more polluted than outdoor air, and also noted that Americans spend 90 percent of their time indoors. All of the indoor air pollutants listed in Table 1 have been shown to be harmful to the respiratory tract.

Sick building syndrome, or SBS, is an unscientific term used to describe a pattern of disease symptoms linked to poor indoor air quality in workplaces, schools, homes, and other buildings. A "sick building" is one in which 20 percent or more of the occupants experience discomfort traceable to contaminated indoor air. Nationwide, as many as 80 million buildings may be affected. Nearly a fifth of the workforce in the United States has reported indoor air pollution ailments, ranging from headaches and fatigue to colds, influenza, and long-term respiratory illnesses (e.g., chronic sinusitis, chronic bronchitis). The annual cost in sick days and medical expenses is estimated to be $3 billion.

The EPA's own building in Washington, D.C., ironically

serves as an excellent example of SBS. For several years, more than a thousand of the 5500 employees at EPA headquarters are known to have had significant health complaints. They have included headaches, rashes, nausea, fatigue, blurred vision, chills, sneezing, fever, irritability, forgetfulness, hoarseness, dizziness, and burning sensations in their throats, ears, eyes, and chests. One employee commented, "I was afraid I was going to die in the place." Several of these symptoms can be attributed to sick sinuses and chronically inflamed respiratory tracts.

Table 1.
INDOOR AIR POLLUTANTS

Combustion Products
   Tobacco smoke
   Coal- or wood-burning fireplaces and stoves
   Fuel combustion gases from gas-fired appliances such as
      ranges, clothes dryers, water heaters, and fireplaces;
      they produce nitrogen dioxide, carbon monoxide,
      nitrous oxides, sulfur oxides, hydrocarbons, and
      formaldehyde
Particulates (these are mostly from outdoor air)
   Dust
   Pollen
   Particles (frayed materials)
   Asbestos in ceilings
Chemicals and Chemical Solutions (chemicals that affect
      indoor air quality are those associated with architecture,
      the interior, artifacts, and maintenance)
   Fungicides and pesticides in carpet-cleaning residues and
      sprays
   Formaldehyde used in the manufacture of insulation,
      plywood, fiberboard, furniture, and wood paneling
   Toxic solvents in oil-based paints, finishes, coatings, and
      wall sealants
   Aerosol sprays

Table 1 (cont'd.)

Office equipment chemicals; those used with photocopiers and computers are common offenders, causing chronic headaches and fatigue

Microorganisms* (primarily from humidifiers, air conditioners, and any other building components affected by excessive moisture)
Bacteria
Viruses
Molds; these are most prevalent in excessively humid climates and are a primary cause of sinus problems in these areas (e.g., Florida and the Gulf Coast states)
Dust mites

Radionuclides*
Radon, a radioactive gas emitted from the earth that enters homes primarily through basements, crawl spaces, and water supply (especially from wells); it can attach to the particulates of cigarette smoke, dust particles, and natural aerosols

Automotive Fumes
Sources include outdoor traffic, outdoor parking lots, and outdoor loading and unloading spaces, as well as indoor garages

Odors
Those emanating from smoke, fragrances, molds, pollen, and chemicals can contribute most to sinus, allergy, and respiratory problems

---

* These are responsible for the majority of the significant health problems.

A major explanation for the syndrome, experts say, is the nationwide campaign to conserve energy after the energy crisis of the mid-1970s by sealing and insulating buildings. The "tight," energy-efficient homes and buildings that evolved have a relatively low energy demand, but a correspondingly low ventilation rate. The demise of the operable-window building and the replacement of natural ventilation with mechanical ventilation have diminished the flow of fresh air, trapping pollutants inside. Furthermore, the fresh air in most cities, as you've just learned, is anything but fresh. There has also been an increase in the use of energy-conserving heating and air conditioning systems, which has often led to increased circulation of polluted indoor air. Another factor in the deterioration of indoor air quality is the type of materials used to construct and furnish buildings. Nonpolluting natural materials and fibers are now seldom used. Instead, buildings and furniture are made of petrochemical-based products and materials that can emit harmful chemical vapors over long periods of time.

As for the EPA and its sick headquarters, after the expenditure of hundreds of thousands of dollars to try to solve the problem, the symptoms continue. I would say to the EPA, "Protector, protect thyself."

There is, in fact, a great deal that can be done to improve indoor air quality. Chapter 8 explores some of the possibilities for improving indoor air quality.

DRY AIR

An important function of the sinuses is to humidify the air we breathe; a person with weak sinuses may therefore have a problem in situations with an abundance of dry air. Moist air (between 40 and 60 percent humidity) is very helpful for the proper functioning of the mucous membrane, especially the cilia. Although usually synonymous with hot air, dry air occurs in conjunction with other phenomena as well. Dry air is associated with

— arid or semiarid climate
— forced hot air heating systems; they not only dry, but give the sinuses more filtering to do
— air conditioning, especially in cars
— oxygen therapy for various respiratory conditions
— wind
— mountains: the higher the elevation, the drier the air
— wood-burning stoves, the most drying of all

Dry air is hard on sinuses, but very moist air can also cause problems. Many microorganisms, i.e., bacteria, viruses, and molds, thrive when the humidity exceeds 60 percent.

COLD AIR

Although the moisture content of cold air is generally much higher than that of dry air, the shock of cold temperatures to the mucous membrane of an impaired sinus can cause significant irritation and ciliary injury, and often results in at least a runny nose. The healthiest air is between 65° and 85°F.

ALLERGIES

People who have nasal allergies (hay fever) and asthma are very susceptible to sinus infections. The same basic process takes place as I have previously described with the common cold and cigarette smoke. The nasal and sinus mucosa are extremely sensitive, i.e., hyperactive and potentially hypersecretory. When an allergic reaction takes place there is swelling of the mucosa and obstruction of the sinuses.

Many people claim they are "allergic" to cigarette smoke, or dust, or some other irritant in the air. Most of the time they are not really describing an allergy, but an extreme irritation of the mucous membrane. This sensitivity causes a similar end result in the nose, stuffiness and mucus drainage, but the process is a bit different. Actual nasal allergies are usually caused by airborne pollen from grass, trees, weeds, flowers, molds, and animal dander (cats, dogs, horses, etc.). In many areas of the United States, these allergies are the major contributors to sinus problems. However, be aware that often the individual complaining of a "year-round allergy problem" may have chronic sinusitis.

In recent years an increasing number of physicians have become nutrition oriented and are recognizing that food allergies may be an important factor in causing chronic sinusitis. The foods most often implicated are wheat, cow's milk and all dairy products, chocolate, corn, soy, white sugar, yeast (brewer's and bakers'), oranges, tomatoes, bell peppers, white potatoes, eggs, garlic, peanuts, black pepper, red meat, coffee, black tea, beer, wine, and champagne. Sensitivities usually comprise all foods with these ingredients.

OCCUPATIONAL HAZARDS

A job that involves any of the aforementioned factors—any type of dirty, dry, extremely hot, or extremely cold air—would be considered a high risk to the sinuses. In my experience, those at highest risk include

— auto mechanics
— construction workers (especially carpenters, who are also the highest risk group for ethmoid sinus cancer in the United States)
— painters
— beauticians
— airport and airline personnel (mechanics, maintenance workers, baggage handlers, flight attendants, and even pilots)
— white-collar workers in offices where there are one or more smokers
— policemen
— firemen
— parking garage attendants
— professional cyclists (the highest risk group; they have more air to filter and are exposed to extremely cold, dry, and often dirty air)*

DENTAL PROBLEMS

After birth, the roots of the teeth and the maxillary sinus come into close proximity; at times they are separated only by paper-thin bone or sinus mucosa. Because of this proximity, periapical abscesses or periodontitis of the upper teeth may extend into the sinus cavity and cause maxillary sinusitis. Minor trauma or injury, dental instrumentation, extraction, or displacement of a chronically inflamed tooth can lead to perforation of the sinus cavity.

The incidence of dental-related sinusitis in children is un-

* When I worked as the team physician for the 7-Eleven cycling team during the 1986 Coors International Bicycle Classic, a total of five riders in the competition, including Eric Heiden of 7-Eleven, had to drop out due to sinus infections—this in spite of the fact that professional cyclists are the most physically fit human beings I have ever known.

known but probably significant, particularly in adolescents. In adults, possibly 10 percent of maxillary sinus infections are thought to be of dental origin.

IMMUNODEFICIENCY

The immune system is the human body's natural defender against infection, cancer, or inflammation—any form of illness. In some people, for reasons medical science has been unable to explain, the immune system does not function normally. A vital component of this system are proteins called immunoglobulins that fight infection. In immunodeficiency there is a decrease in the amount of one or two of these proteins. This condition can be diagnosed by a blood test. Most often there is no known cause, but some people have a hereditary predisposition, are on a cancer chemotherapy treatment program, or may be taking cortisone long-term for a chronic condition. Although this is just beginning to be recognized as a possible cause by medical science, I have been observing for quite some time that people who have had long-term or repeated courses of antibiotic therapy appear to have a very weak immune system. They are extremely prone to recurrent sinus infections.

MALFORMATIONS

Malformations include any physical problem that would result in the obstruction of the tiny sinus openings, the ostia. The most common malformations are deviated septum (the wall that divides the two sides of the nose), enlarged adenoids (especially in young children), polyps, cysts, or turbinate hypertrophy (swelling of the mucosal lining covering the internal nasal ridges).

EMOTIONAL STRESS

Emotional stress is probably the single most important determinant in whether someone develops a sinus infection. All the other factors I have described in this chapter have the *potential* for adversely affecting the sinuses. But what is it that triggers that potential? Why is it that a person with weak sinuses can be exposed to the same "risky" conditions many times but only occasionally develops a sinus infection? I am convinced that stress is usually the answer.

In the past few years, psychoneuroimmunology, the science of mind/body medicine, has been the subject of much discussion in the medical community. Through this field there is emerging a wealth of information on the profound impact that our thoughts, beliefs, feelings, and attitudes have upon the functioning of our body's immune system and on our total state of health. This knowledge is implemented in holistic medicine, and its application to the treatment of sinus disease will be discussed in Part II.

Chapter 3

Recognizing a Sick Sinus: Acute and Chronic

Throughout this book I use the term "sinusitis" to refer to sinus problems in general. This word actually means "inflammation of a sinus" and encompasses two distinctly different medical diagnoses: acute sinusitis and chronic sinusitis.

ACUTE SINUSITIS

Acute sinusitis is another way of saying "sinus infection." This is the problem that usually requires medical attention. I've already mentioned that the common cold is most often the cause of a sinus infection, so let's look at this a bit more closely.

Usually the person who's had negligible previous sinus problems will notice that his cold just won't quit after about seven to ten days; or that the symptoms of the cold have actually gotten much worse; or that the cold was almost gone for one to two weeks and now it's back again. After close questioning it's apparent that the "cold" never really went away.

In people with already weak sinuses (caused by previous sinus infections), the common cold usually results in problems occurring much sooner. They might notice the typical symptoms of a sinus infection arising in only two to three days. The underlying condition of the sinuses will usually determine how soon the symptoms appear. The important thing to keep in mind is that a common cold very often precedes the onset of acute sinusitis. Its presence somewhere in the story of one's illness will help in the recognition of a sick sinus.

What else are we looking for? Are these symptoms different

for adults than for children (under the age of twelve)? The answer to the latter question is yes. The most common symptoms are as follows, with the first four being present in almost every adult case of a sinus infection.

HEAD CONGESTION

Most people describe this symptom as "fullness" or "a stuffy head." The nose may or may not be stuffy as well. This symptom is most obvious in the morning upon arising from bed. It is often relieved, although not eliminated, by a hot shower. One may also notice that voice, smell, and taste are somewhat altered. These symptoms, however, are more subtle than the primary one of head congestion. There is a very definite awareness of a fullness in the head or a dull ache behind or above the eyes. If present, it's quite obvious. "Dizziness" and "lightheadedness" are other words that might be used to describe this symptom.

HEADACHE AND FACIAL PAIN

I've combined these two because it's often difficult to differentiate between them. With acute sinusitis, pain and sometimes swelling will occur in the region of the affected sinus (Figure D). This usually results from air, pus, and mucus being trapped within the obstructed sinus. An infected maxillary sinus will cause pain in the cheek (sometimes swelling too), under the eye, and/or in the teeth of the upper jaw, particularly the molars. At times, the tooth pain may be so severe as to prompt a visit to the dentist. When air is prevented from entering a sinus by a swollen mucous membrane at the opening, a vacuum can be created, also resulting in severe pain in the affected sinus.

Infected ethmoid sinuses produce pain between and behind the eyes, and tenderness when pressure is applied to the sides of the nose; frontals, in the forehead and over the eyes; and sphenoids, a generalized pain, deep in the head, which becomes aggravated whenever your head is jarred (as when your heel strikes hard against the ground in walking). Sphenoid pain can often be present as a headache in the back of the head at the base of the skull.

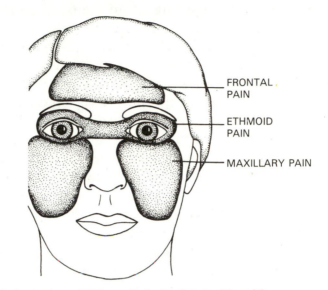

FRONTAL PAIN

ETHMOID PAIN

MAXILLARY PAIN

Figure D. Location of Sinus Pain in Acute Sinusitis.

Children may have facial pain accompanied by swelling of the orbit of the eye that involves the upper eyelid, lower lid, or both. Gradual in onset, the swelling is most obvious in the early morning shortly after arising. The swelling may decrease or even disappear during the day, only to reappear the following day. Children may also experience photophobia, which is an unwillingness to open their eyes in bright light.

I should note that some of the most incapacitating headaches I've encountered have resulted from infected frontal sinuses. Sinus headaches tend to worsen when you bend your head forward or lie down. Hence, they often feel worse in the morning after you've lain in bed for hours, and ease somewhat later in the day.

EXTREME FATIGUE

There is hardly a sick patient I can think of who doesn't complain of some degree of fatigue. Most people, even if they're not ill, would admit to being tired for some part of the day. Therefore, I'd like to emphasize the word "extreme," and note that I'm talking about a definite change in normal energy level.

In addition to inquiring about the nasal and head symptoms that are usually mentioned by the patient, I always ask the question, "Does your whole body feel sick in some way?" or "Do you feel especially tired?" The answer is frequently yes. This fatigue illustrates the point that acute sinusitis is usually a systemic illness, i.e., one that affects the entire being. These people are sick all over. The medical term that best describes this phenomenon is "malaise," meaning a feeling of general discomfort. It's often accompanied by significant irritability. But in addition to this feeling, people with sinus infections usually are sleeping more at night, having some difficulty getting through a full day at work, or perhaps even taking unaccustomed naps. In people who exercise regularly, the change in energy level will be even more evident.

At times, fatigue may even be patients' chief complaint. The bad cold that they had was as long ago as two or three months, and "I just haven't been myself since." These people do not come in complaining of the cold that they still have. Most of the time they think they're finished with it. But in fact, if asked, they'll admit to a stuffy head in the morning and occasional yellow mucus that they have to spit out. These patients pose a tough diagnostic challenge to the physician, as some of them have been tired for so long they have no recollection of any physical illness. I have seen them frequently misdiagnosed with anything from depression to menopause. A few days of antibiotics, however, can do what months of estrogen was unable to do.

YELLOW MUCUS

This is the question that seems to make patients most uncomfortable: "What color is your mucus?" The usual response, accompanied by a grimace, is, "Eww, I never look at it!" I ask this question for two locations—the nose, and more importantly, the back of the throat. The classic presentation of acute sinusitis, which one usually does not see in an adult, is yellow (actually a yellow/green) mucus coming from one nostril. Children with a sinus infection usually have this colored mucus running from their nose. However, if it's not (no pun intended), it can sometimes make the diagnosis difficult, since most kids are not great nose-blowers. Sniffing actually makes matters worse, since it tends to suck bacteria into the sinus. I usually try to have young patients blow their nose in the exam room, while I'm there. If you are checking your child at home, please remember to use white tissues; yellow won't help at all. Sinusitis is so often missed in children that in a recent article in a pediatric journal, it was stated that almost 25 percent of all diagnosed upper respiratory tract infections (the common cold) in kids were actually cases of acute sinusitis.

In adults, if it's yellow from the nose, that will help in making the diagnosis. But in many cases it is either clear or white mucus, or there is no mucus at all from the nose. It seems that in most cases of acute sinusitis, the infected or yellow mucus drains down the back of the throat. People are most aware of this in the morning, when they get out of bed and spit into the sink some of the mucus they've collected during the night. This first morning mucus specimen is helpful in making the diagnosis, but it can be present without acute sinusitis. Therefore, the most important question I ask an adult is, "Are you spitting out yellow mucus during the rest of the day, other than first thing in the morning?" Unfortunately, most people will respond with "I swallow it," or "It's not convenient to spit it out," or the old standby, "I never look at it!" If I'm still suspicious of a sinus infection, then I'll ask if they're even aware of mucus dripping down the back of the throat. If they're not aware of this occurring during the day, then I'll go back to "How about when you wake up in the morning?" Often I'll see patients who aren't aware of mucus drainage, but when I look at their throat, there is a thick yellow band of mucus coming down from their sinuses.

I've spent a lot of time on this topic not because I enjoy discussing "gross" subjects, as my daughter Julie would say, but because it is extremely helpful in making the diagnosis. There are very few objective physical signs of acute sinusitis, and this one is consistently present.

REFINING THE DIAGNOSIS
Most ENT (ear, nose, and throat) specialists would find

yellow mucus to be too indefinite a finding with which to make a diagnosis. Until 1986, they usually attempted to confirm the diagnosis with a sinus X-ray. However, the X-ray costs about $40 (more than most office visits to a family doctor or pediatrician) and it is extremely unreliable (often people will have every symptom of a sinus infection and the X-ray will be normal); thus it is impractical at best.

In the past several years, new technology has made the definitive diagnosis of acute sinusitis much more feasible. The CT ("cat") scan, a computerized tomographic X-ray technique, has been able to show areas of the sinuses never clearly visible with conventional sinus X-rays. As a result, the diagnosis of sinus disease and hence the statistics on its incidence have risen dramatically in many medical practices since 1986. Unfortunately, the average sinus CT scan costs at least $130.

To help reduce medical costs, as well as to assist primary care physicians, allergists, and ENT specialists in treating sinus infections, it would be a great advantage to have a generally accepted clinical diagnosis of acute sinusitis. This is what I am attempting to present—a list of signs and symptoms that are so often present with sinus infections that they will preclude the need for X-rays and other expensive diagnostic procedures in making the diagnosis. Ultimately, this knowledge will expedite the treatment of this most common malady.

The picture presented by acute sinusitis can vary greatly—some people are very sick, others minimally uncomfortable. But you can usually depend on these elements to make a definitive clinical diagnosis in an *adult:* a preceding cold, head congestion, headache, extreme fatigue, and postnasal yellow mucus. In a *child* the most common symptoms are nasal yellow mucus, fever, foul-smelling breath, and cough.

MORE DIAGNOSTIC CLUES

The following symptoms are not quite as consistent as these first ones, but are frequently present.

Fever

This is much more common in children than adults. When

it's present in an adult, it's usually low-grade (less than 101° F). However, it's not uncommon to see kids run high fevers (103° to 105° F) with acute sinusitis. Often it's early in the course of the infection, and other symptoms are not yet obvious, making the diagnosis difficult. The point here is that because fever accompanies so many different infections, it can't be considered an important diagnostic symptom. However, if I'm suspicious of sinusitis, fever can be a helpful sign in confirming the diagnosis along with the other symptoms that are present.

Nasal Congestion and Rhinorrhea

This simply means a stuffy and runny nose. We already know that these are the primary symptoms of the common cold and that a cold usually precedes acute sinusitis. Therefore, it's quite common to have an overlapping of the two infections. The important things to keep in mind are that, in adults, stuffiness is more prominent with sinusitis than the runny nose, and it is often present on only one side of the nose. With children the yellow nasal discharge can be copious. Also, with a cold, draining mucus is usually clear and/or white and thin and/or watery, while with sinusitis it's usually thick and yellow.

Sore Throat

This is probably the most common complaint in any family doctor's office. There are a variety of causes, but a substantial number of sore throats result from postnasal mucus drainage down the back of the throat and from mouth breathing. When this occurs, it does not always mean the underlying problem is sinusitis, but there are a few key points to investigate to find out if it is. A sore throat from sinusitis is usually not consistent throughout the day—it is much worse in the morning upon awakening. In fact, the sore throat itself can keep people from sleeping through the night. This is the result of the constant postnasal mucus drainage from the sinuses and mouth breathing subsequent to a stuffy nose. The dry air most of us breathe at night in our bedrooms can be very irritating. Once I've established that the sore throat is much worse first thing in the morning, the next step is to determine if there is any awareness of mucus draining down the back of the throat. In children, this drainage often results in bad breath. From that point I merely have to run through a checklist of the other potential sinus symptoms—mucus color, recent cold, fatigue, fever, etc.—to determine if this is sinusitis or something else. Most of these questions would be asked anyway as part of a thorough investigation of any sore throat.

Laryngitis

Laryngitis (hoarseness) is another common symptom of a sinus infection. It results from the same factors that cause sore throat, primarily postnasal mucus draining down into the larynx, causing irritation, inflammation, and swelling of the vocal cords and the arytenoid cartilages in the larynx.

Cough

I am sure that the chief complaints of cough and sore throat account for the bulk of the patients who come to a family doctor's office with a sinus infection. These are the symptoms that result in the greatest discomfort and the most loss of sleep. Unfortunately, they are also the symptoms that result in the highest number of misdiagnoses. A cough is often mistakenly thought to be bronchitis. Why? Because the cough of a sinusitis results from the same thing that causes the sore throat—yellow mucus draining down the back of the throat and continuing into the trachea or upper airway. Most physicians are aware that a productive (mucus-producing) cough that brings up a purulent or yellow mucus is often bronchitis. It isn't unusual to make that diagnosis in spite of hearing clear lungs with the stethoscope. So it's easy to understand this common mistake. But it's just as easy to ask a few simple questions to rule out bronchitis and rule in acute sinusitis.

The cough of a sinus infection in adults is often worse as soon as they lie down in bed at night. It isn't usually too bad during the day when they're upright. In children it tends to be more persistent throughout the day. We tend to swallow the postnasal mucus drainage, consciously or (usually) unconsciously, while we're up and about. This gets the mucus away from the trachea and into the stomach. (Swallowing the mucus can result in another not-uncommon symptom with sinus infections: gastrointestinal upset, i.e., abdominal discomfort and/or loose bowels. There may be two or three loosish bowel movements per day—not quite diarrhea, but a definite change in one's bowel pattern. This isn't nearly as common as the other symptoms I've mentioned, so I apologize for getting off the tract—respiratory, that is. Now, back to the cough.)

After asking about the timing of the cough, I usually want to know, "Does the cough feel like it's deep in your chest or does it feel more like a tickle in the back of your throat?" The latter, a drier cough, is much more typical of sinusitis, while the former, a wet mucusy cough, is more indicative of bronchitis. In the past few years, I've noticed a definite increase in the number of patients who are infected in both the sinuses and the lungs simultaneously. Medicine calls this sinobronchitis. If the antibiotic treatments for sinusitis and bronchitis were the same, there would be no great necessity to differentiate between the two. However, this is not the case, and I believe it is valuable to be as specific as possible in a treatment program.

I began this chapter by describing acute sinusitis as an infection usually requiring medical attention. A visit to the doctor has a twofold purpose—to diagnose the problem and to begin treating it. Ideally, there should also be a third objective—education and prevention, i.e., teaching the patient how to care for his sinuses so effectively that he can avoid any future office visits for the same problem. However, the feasibility of attaining this lofty goal in the midst of a busy practice has so far eluded me. It is from that frustration that the desire to write this book began.

As one can easily understand from reading this chapter, the recognition of acute sinusitis is not a simple matter, even for physicians. This chapter and the next should be referred to frequently. For those who are plagued with repeated sinus infections, you'll be surprised at how quickly and easily this new knowledge is absorbed.

CHRONIC SINUSITIS

For those of you who thought "acute" was no problem, perhaps I'll be able to challenge you with chronic sinusitis. This is the diagnosis believed by the National Center for Health Statistics to be the most common chronic disease in the United States. Yet, although it affects nearly one out of every seven Americans, many who have it couldn't tell you, and doctors have even more difficulty with this diagnosis than with acute sinusitis. The situation is similar to that of the hundreds of thousands of people who have high blood pressure and diabetes, which are other common chronic conditions, and are not aware of it. Although they may not be able to attach a label to it, what these sinus sufferers are very familiar with are postnasal drip, congestion, headaches, fatigue, halitosis, weak sense of smell, and Kleenex. These nuisances have been a part of their daily lives for years and something most have just accepted. Doctors haven't paid much attention to chronic sinusitis because they don't consider it a significant disease, i.e., one that could shorten your life expectancy.

Chronic sinusitis can be either a persistent, low-grade infection or a chronic inflammation of the mucosal lining of the nose and sinus cavities. In the former category I am seeing an increasing number of moderately to severely afflicted patients (I'll call them group 1) who have taken repeated courses of antibiotics (often for more than a year) and/or have had sinus surgery, with no significant positive effect. These are extremely frustrated and often angry individuals, whose physicians share their exasperation. Medical science has done all it can do, and to no avail.

There is another group—group 2—of chronically infected people who have accepted their long-term (often lifelong) condition as something they must live with. They were either told this by a physician following an unsuccessful attempt at treatment or have just been unaware that they even had a medically treatable problem. Their infection usually persists in a low-grade state without becoming incapacitating. These people don't feel sick and have adjusted to their condition as their normal state of health. Group 2 is similar to group 3, who have chronic inflammation without infection. Inflammation involves pain, swelling, and increased secretions from the mucous membrane, but without the causative agents of bacteria, viruses, or fungi that are present in infection. People with infection are usually sicker and weaker and have a somewhat depressed immune system.

The degree of discomfort is generally much less for groups 2 and 3 than it is for group 1, but each group shares the following symptoms: head and/or nasal congestion; nasal and postnasal mucus drainage (often yellow in groups 1 and 2, white in group 3); headaches, irritability, and fatigue (especially in group 1); halitosis; and a diminished sense of smell and taste. Most of these chronic sinus sufferers have an increased sensitivity to all of the factors mentioned in Chapter 2—smoke, pollution, pollen, dryness, cold, fumes, etc. The more they are exposed to any one of these irritants, the more pronounced the symptoms will be and the more often these people may develop acute sinus infections. For many, a routine common cold has become a rare occurrence. What starts out that way frequently develops into an acute sinusitis. In fact, almost any infection, whether it begins as influenza, strep throat, gastroenteritis (vomiting and diarrhea), or a number of others, will often indirectly cause a sinus infection just by depressing an already weakened immune system. (Chronic infection decreases one's natural resistance.)

The recognition and diagnosis of chronic sinusitis is difficult. Until recently it has been based almost entirely on the patient's description of his condition—the medical history. An X-ray might reveal a thickened mucosa, but this is not necessarily diagnostic of sinusitis. In a small percentage of cases a doctor's examination might show a deviated nasal septum or polyps that could have blocked the sinus openings, the ostia, contributing to the onset of chronic sinusitis. In the past few years, medical technology has developed a telescope-like device called an endoscope. This flexible fiber optic instrument can be inserted into the nose for a much clearer view of the areas of possible sinus blockage. It can not only help to confirm the diagnosis of chronic sinusitis but has been responsible for greatly improving the results of sinus surgery (see Chapter 6).

The vast majority of chronic sinus sufferers recognize that something isn't right in their nose and sinuses but aren't sure of the exact diagnosis. For most, the condition began as a result of one or more episodes of acute sinusitis, repeated nasal allergies, or constant exposure to irritants such as cigarette smoke, pollution, fumes, etc. These factors can all leave the sinuses in a permanently damaged state. This is not a directly life-threatening illness. But it certainly poses a threat to the health of our lungs, affects us daily, and is an energy-draining condition that can have a profound impact on our ability to fully enjoy our lives.

Chapter 4

Treating Acute Sinusitis

What does it mean to "treat" an ailment? It usually depends upon what the condition is. In some instances treatment implies cure, with the expectation that the problem will never recur. These treatments are most often surgical, e.g., appendicitis is treated with an appendectomy.

At other times, to treat means to improve symptoms of a condition that has no known cure. This could involve anything from cancer and AIDS to the common cold and sore throat. This category of treatment comprises the bulk of a physician's livelihood—almost 75 percent of all ailments fall into this treatment realm.

Acute sinusitis is a bacterial infection in one or more of the sinus cavities. The goal of treatment in this case is to kill the bacteria, open the blocked sinus duct, and restore the mucus/cilia cleansing system, while relieving all of the possible symptoms discussed in the last chapter. This type of treatment differs from the first two I mentioned. Acute sinusitis is an infection that does have a cure, but the chances of its recurring at some point, either months or years later, are very high.

Acute sinusitis is not a simple infection to treat, such as strep throat would be. The bacteria that cause the infection are not often identified. An antibiotic is selected based upon the bacteria most likely to cause the infection. The antibiotic is taken by mouth and absorbed into the bloodstream. But because of the relatively poor blood supply in the sinuses, it usually takes several days before the effect of the drug is felt, especially in adults. For this reason, strong antibiotics in relatively high dosages taken for long periods of time are often required to treat this infection.

The next objective is to open the blocked sinus duct and the ostium so that the infected mucus can drain from the sinus. The type of drug that best accomplishes the opening of the duct is a decongestant, since it shrinks the swollen mucous membrane. However, most decongestants also have a drying effect, especially if used in combination with an antihistamine. (Most commercial decongestants contain an antihistamine.) This drying will thicken the mucus and prevent it from draining.

Acute sinusitis is an infection without an accepted standard treatment program. Antibiotics have been, and continue to be, the primary component of the traditional medical treatment. However, if there was one drug that always worked for everyone, this would be a very brief discussion and I would not have to devote an entire chapter to the subject. The reality is that treatment of acute sinusitis can vary with each individual patient and with the physician who is administering the treatment. During the past decade, physicians have had to employ greater creativity, using a vastly expanded arsenal of antibiotics, decongestants, expectorants, nasal sprays, and antitussives to succeed in treating sinus infections.

ANTIBIOTICS

The bacteria most often responsible for causing sinus infections in both adults and children are *Streptococcus pneumoniae* and *Hemophilus influenzae*. Recently there has been a marked increase in the incidence of *Staphylococcus aureus,* especially in children, perhaps because of improved diagnostic techniques.

Unfortunately, the only antibiotics that are effective in treating all the bacteria that cause sinusitis are quite expensive. As sinus infections become more difficult to treat, especially those caused by *Staphylococcus aureus,* medical science continues to come to the rescue with more powerful antibiotics.

For the past decade the first drug of choice has been ampicillin or its counterpart, amoxicillin. The dosage of amoxicillin is either 250 or 500 mg (125 or 250 mg in children) three times a day (every eight hours). Both are taken for ten days. This is a routine first step, but it is a hefty dose of antibiotic! Adult patients are instructed that they will notice definite improvement and that the yellow mucus will start to clear in about four to five days. In children the response is usually faster, with fever, nasal drainage, and cough markedly reduced after about forty-eight hours. Patients are told to be sure to take the medicine for the entire ten days. Often the infection will remain if this instruction is not followed. Many physicians now routinely treat with amoxicillin for fourteen days instead of ten, to reduce the number of treatment failures. Fortunately, for the majority of patients with acute sinusitis, a ten-day course of amoxicillin is all they'll need.

In spite of their compliance with instructions, about 5 to 10 percent of patients will return or call shortly after the ten days, still complaining of most of their symptoms. Some will report that they felt much better while on the antibiotic, but that as soon as they stopped taking it, the symptoms recurred. Others will tell me they experienced no improvement whatsoever, and usually in a tone of voice that conveys the very clear message, "You'd better get rid of this infection real fast." These are not my most pleasant patients. Nor should they be. They've usually had the sinusitis for at least three weeks and have now made their second visit to the doctor.

With my second attempt at treatment, I'll almost always choose a different antibiotic. The second-choice antibiotics have a bit broader spectrum of efficacy than amoxicillin; all of them are more expensive. Table 2 lists both amoxicillin and the second-step drugs that are commonly used for the treatment of acute sinusitis.

Most physicians have their own favorite second-step antibiotic, one with which they've had the most therapeutic success with the fewest unpleasant side effects. Ceclor has been replaced by Ceftin as the popular choice. Both of them cost about $50 for a ten-day supply, but Ceftin seems to be more effective. It can be given twice a day in a strength equivalent to Ceclor given three times per day and is easily absorbed with food.

A small but growing percentage of patients are still not cured following a ten-day course of a second-step antibiotic, or the infection returns shortly after they finish the antibiotic. These

Table 2.
ANTIBIOTICS FOR ACUTE SINUSITIS

Brand Name & Quantity	Generic Equivalent	Strength/Average Dose	Adults (12 + yr.) or Children	Average Price
	Amoxicillin Capsules #30	1) 250 mg 1 3X/day 2) 500 mg for 10 days	1) children 2) adults	1) $7 2) $9
	Amoxicillin Suspension 150 cc	250 mg/5cc (1 tsp.) 3X/dX10d	children	$7
Ceclor Capsules #30		250 mg 1 3X/dX10d		$48
Ceclor Suspension 150 cc		250 mg/5 cc 3X/dX10d	children	$41
Bactrim DS #20 or Septra DS	Trimethoprim-Sulfamethoxazole	1 2X/dX10d	adults	$22 $10 (generic)
Bactrim Suspension 200 cc	Trimethoprim-Sulfamethoxazole	10 cc (2 tsp) 2X/dX10d	children	$17 $ 9 (generic)
Vibramycin or Vibra-Tabs #20	Doxycycline	100 mg 1 2X/dX10d	adults	$56 $12 (generic)
Pediazole Suspension 200 cc	Erythromycin-Sulfisoxazole	5 cc 4X/dX10d	children	$26 $17 (generic)
Ceftin Tablets #20		250 mg 1 2X/dX10d	adults	$50
Cipro Tablets #20		500 mg 1 2X/dX10d	adults	$50
Suprax Tablets #10		400 mg 1X/dX10d	adults	$48
Suprax Suspension 100 cc		100 mg/5cc 1X/dX10d	children	$44

patients are good candidates for further diagnostic evaluation with an X-ray, CT scan, or rhinolaryngoscopy to see if there is a structural obstruction of the sinus. It sometimes helps to take a two- or even three-week course of the antibiotic and gradually taper it off over the last five to seven days. This seems to allow the body's immune system a better chance to take over for the antibiotic. Whatever the reason, this strategy does appear to be more effective than abruptly stopping the drug a patient has been taking for two to three weeks.

During the past year, I have seen several new patients for acute and chronic sinusitis with a history of having taken nearly consecutive courses of different antibiotics for almost two years. It's true that these are extreme cases, but it appears that many physicians are being confronted with such problems. Since the first edition of *Sinus Survival* was published in November 1988, three new "big gun" antibiotics have begun to be used commonly as a last resort with stubborn sinus infections. They are Ceftin, Cipro, and Suprax (ineffective against *Staphylococcus*). Their efficacy has been impressive—but how long can we continue to rely upon the development of ever more powerful drugs?

DECONGESTANTS AND EXPECTORANTS

The decongestants are specifically used to open the ostia and sinus ducts while relieving the symptoms of head and nasal congestion, headache, facial pain, and to some extent, sore throat and cough. Expectorants, which are mucus thinners, can help to relieve the same symptoms.

As I've already mentioned, the challenge of using a decongestant in the treatment of acute sinusitis is to find one whose benefits outweigh the side effects. Decongestants are readily available in many familiar over-the-counter (OTC) products, e.g., Dristan, Contac, Allerest, Drixoral, Actifed, Dimetapp, Triaminicin, and a host of other "cold remedies." However, every one of these has an antihistamine in combination with the decongestant. This is also true of Sinutab and many other "sinus remedies." Given the drying effect of antihistamines and the subsequent thickening of the mucus as a result of this drying, I'm convinced they do more harm than good. They're fine if all you're trying to treat is a cold. But in many instances, I believe they've actually helped a cold progress into a sinus infection. So, if you have a history of sinus problems, I would advise you to avoid taking an antihistamine. If you're not sure about the ingredients of an OTC product, ask the pharmacist.

The most common ingredients in both prescription (Rx) and OTC decongestants are pseudoephedrine, phenylpropanolamine, and phenylephrine. Each of these chemicals works similarly in shrinking swollen mucous membranes to reduce nasal and sinus congestion. Many products contain these decongestants in combination—some (available only by prescription) include two of these ingredients, others only one, along with an analgesic (pain reliever) or an expectorant or an antitussive (cough suppressant).

At the pharmacy there is a myriad of choices. I will attempt to give you a "map" to lead you through the maze of cold and sinus preparations. Before you begin the process, it would be helpful to ask yourself, "What is it that I'm treating?" What are the symptoms that are most troubling you? Are you really stuffed up? Or is it the headache, the cough, the sore throat, or the thick mucus that you'd most like to eliminate? Since it's usually more than one of these symptoms, you'll probably be looking for a medication that has a decongestant in combination with something else (but not with an antihistamine). Those that I recommend are found in Tables 3 through 7. If all you need is a plain decongestant, then Sudafed tablets are an excellent choice. If you have a lot of thick mucus draining, don't want a decongestant, and would just like to have an expectorant, then Fenesin and Organidin are both good prescription drugs.

Table 3.
DECONGESTANTS WITH ANALGESICS (OTC)

Allerest No Drowsiness Tablets
Coldrine Tablets
Congesprin Cold Tablets for Children
Dristan Maximum Strength Caplets
Dristan Sinus Tablets
Fiogesic Tablets
Naldegesic Tablets
Ornex Caplets
St. Joseph Cold Tablets for Children
Sinarest No Drowsiness Tablets
Sine-Aid Maximum Strength Caplets
Sine-Aid Sinus Headache Tablets
Sine-Off Maximum Strength No Drowsiness Formula Caplets
Sinus Excedrin Tablets and Caplets
Sinutab Maximum Strength Without Drowsiness Caplets
Spec-T Sore Throat/Decongestant Lozenges
Sudafed Maximum Strength Sinus Tablets and Caplets
Super Anahist Tablets
Tylenol Maximum Strength Sinus Tablets and Caplets

Table 4.
DECONGESTANTS WITH EXPECTORANTS (OTC)

Robitussin PE Syrup
Triaminic Expectorant

Table 5.
DECONGESTANTS WITH EXPECTORANTS (Rx)

Dura-Gest Capsules
Dura-Vent Tablets
Entex Capsules
Entex LA Tablets
Entex Liquid
Guaifed Capsules
Guaifed-PD Capsules
Nolex LA Tablets
Respaire-60 SR Capsules
Respaire-120 SR Capsules
Respinol-LA Tablets
T-Moist Tablets
Tuss-LA Tablets
Zephrex LA Tablets

Tables 3 and 4, and Table 7 in the next section, all list OTC products. Please follow the dosage instructions on the bottle or package. The prescription drugs in Table 5, which your doctor might prescribe, contain the same decongestants and expectorants as those found in the OTC products. The primary difference is that these drugs contain higher doses and are long-acting, continuing to work for up to twelve hours. The exceptions are Entex and Dura-Gest, which is both a brand-name drug and used by most pharmacists as the generic form of Entex. These products are short-acting (can be taken every four to six hours) and contain two decongestants, phenylephrine and phenylpropanolamine, in combination with the expectorant guaifenisen. I find them more effective in the treatment of acute sinusitis than the long-acting preparations. They should be avoided, however, if you have high blood pressure, and they can cause insomnia in adults. (Some young children experience the opposite side effect—drowsiness.) Omitting the bedtime dose usually eliminates the insomnia if it occurs.

I usually don't insist that patients with acute sinusitis take a decongestant as regularly as I do the antibiotic, or for the entire ten-day course. I tell them to take it regularly for the first four to five days, then gradually taper off. If they're still experiencing head and sinus congestion, then they should continue with it. Due to the poor air quality and pressure changes experienced on airplanes, I recommend taking a decongestant during air travel, approximately two hours prior to the scheduled landing time. However, if the flight can be avoided while one still has an active sinus infection, it is advisable to postpone it.

DECONGESTANT SPRAYS

An over-the-counter alternative for those with extreme head and nasal congestion and/or sinus pain is nasal decongestant spray. There are several twelve-hour varieties from which to choose, e.g., Afrin, Dristan, Sinex, Neosynephrin, Vicks. These should be used with great caution and only for two or three days at most. They can easily become addictive! They produce what is called a rebound effect, which means that as their decongestant effect wears off and the head and nasal congestion return, the feeling of stuffiness is worse than it was before using the spray. This elicits a strong desire to spray again, and a vicious circle begins. Be careful with these!

If you've been using a spray regularly and are unable to stop, you'll probably need some help. I would consult with your physician and tell him honestly what's been happening. I've had a high success rate in helping patients to break this habit by using the following regimen:
— Throw away the nasal spray.
— Medrol (generic = methylprednisolone) dosepak 4 mg or prednisone 5 mg; this is a tapered dose of cortisone over a one-week period, and these are prescription drugs.
— Entex or Dura-Gest—a prescription for forty capsules to be taken in a tapered dose (one 3 times/day X 7 days; then one 2 times/day X 7 days; followed by one daily before bed X 7 days) over three weeks.
— Moisture—includes saline nasal spray, ultrasonic humidifier, and steaming in the bathroom (refer to the "Moisture and Irrigation" section in this chapter).
Remember that it is extremely difficult to have healthy sinuses with continued use of a decongestant nasal spray.

Table 6.
ANTITUSSIVES WITH DECONGESTANTS
AND/OR EXPECTORANTS (Rx)

Detussin Expectorant
Donatussin DC Syrup
Hycomine Pediatric Syrup
Hycomine Syrup
Naldecon CX Liquid
Novahistine Expectorant
Nucofed Expectorant
Robitussin A-C
Robitussin-DAC
Triaminic Expectorant with Codeine
Tussend-DAC
Tussend Expectorant
Tussi Organidin
Tussi Organidin DM

ANTITUSSIVES (COUGH SUPPRESSANTS)

If a patient's chief complaint is a cough that's not allowing him to sleep, I'll withhold his bedtime dose of decongestant and substitute a strong prescription cough suppressant containing either codeine or hydrocodone in combination with a decongestant, an expectorant, or both. Such antitussives can cause drowsiness. That's why I rarely recommend them for daytime use. Besides, these people are already tired from having a sinus infection. They don't need any additional sedation. The most commonly prescribed antitussives for sinus patients are listed in Table 6. If a cough suppressant is indicated during the day, especially in children, there are several similar over-the-counter combination drugs from which to choose. They can be taken by both adults and children and are listed in Table 7.

ANALGESICS (PAIN RELIEVERS)

To relieve the frequent symptoms of headache, facial pain, and sore throat, I recommend the over-the-counter pain re-

Table 7.
ANTITUSSIVES WITH DECONGESTANTS AND EXPECTORANTS (OTC)

Ambenyl D Decongestant Formula
Bayer Children's Cough Syrup
Benylin Expectorant Liquid
Cheracol D Cough Liquid
Comtrex Cough Formula
Contac Cough Formula Liquid
Contac Jr. Liquid
Dorcol Children's Cough Syrup
Formula 44D Decongestant Cough Mixture
Formula 44M Liquid
Naldecon DX Pediatric Drops
Naldecon DX Children's Syrup
Naldecon DX Adult Liquid
Naldecon EX Pediatric Drops
Naldecon Senior DX Liquid
Novahistine DXM Syrup
Robitussin-CF
Robitussin DM Cough Calmers Lozenges
Robitussin DM Syrup
Ru-Tuss Expectorant
Sudafed Cough Syrup
Vicks Children's Cough Syrup

lievers Advil or Nuprin. Both contain ibuprofen, which not only relieves pain but also reduces inflammation. To some extent, it can lower a fever. They are dispensed in 200-mg tablets, and it is safe (for adults) to take three or even four of them at a time if the pain is especially severe. This dosage should be taken with food, especially if there is a history of stomach ulcers.

Aspirin has the same effects as ibuprofen but isn't as strong. Tylenol and other acetaminophen-containing products are simply analgesics, with no effect upon the inflamed sinuses. However, if lowering a fever is the primary objective, then both aspirin and Tylenol would be better choices. Any acetaminophen-containing product is the drug of choice for children.

MOISTURE AND IRRIGATION

Moisture helps to empty the sinus of its thick infected mucus and in doing so aids in restoring normal cilial function. As it does this, it also relieves nasal and head congestion, headache, sinus pain, and sore throat. Warm, moist air is best, and the easiest place to get it is in the bathroom. Simply close the door and window and turn on the hot water of the shower to create steam. Then you have the choice of either getting in the shower (after adjusting the temperature, of course) or just sitting and relaxing in the steam until you run out of hot water. Remember to try and make a conscious effort to breathe through your nose, thereby getting the moisture to where it will do the most good. Hot towels applied over the face can also be helpful.

As most of us do not have an endless supply of hot water in our homes, making a steam room of your bathroom can only be done two or three times a day. What about the rest of the time? If you've decided to stay home from work, your best alternative for moist air is an ultrasonic humidifier placed by your bed, with the bedroom door and windows closed. These humidifiers are quiet and very effective in producing a moist environment in an enclosed space. They're available in pharmacies, department stores, and hardware stores in a variety of brand names. The humidifiers' design has not been perfected yet, however. The cool mist ultrasonics put out a fine mineral dust unless distilled water is used to fill them, and the new warm ultrasonics have a tendency to break down. The steam humidifiers or vaporizers can become quite hot, which could be a concern if you have small children. The Bionaire warm ultrasonic humidifier is one that seems to have eliminated most problems. The majority of the room humidifiers cost between $40 and $100. Whatever your choice, be sure the reservoir tank opening is large enough to allow for cleaning, and wipe it out daily with vinegar water. Otherwise it becomes a breeding ground for molds. Whether you're home or not during the day, the humidifier should be used every night while you're treating the sinus infection. The moisture is very helpful in relieving both the cough and sore throat during the night.

I've recently learned from a physician about a product that he's been using for his sinus patients with excellent results. It's called a rhinotherm unit, and it delivers ultrasonically humidified steam directly into the nose. It's made by Twin Med Products in Santa Monica, California, and it sells for $400.

Another simple method for obtaining moisture (assuming your environment is relatively dry, as indoor air tends to be during the winter months in most parts of the United States) is to use a salt water (saline) nasal spray. There are several commercial products available in many pharmacies, e.g., Salinex, Ayr, Ocean, NaSal, and NoseBetter sprays. I am in the process of developing a product called "Sinus Survival Spray." This nonmedicated saline spray will moisten and irrigate as the others do, and the citrus extract it contains will give it the added capability of killing bacteria and viruses in the nose. It should be available by early 1991. You can also make your own saline spray by mixing a teaspoon of salt in a 16-ounce (1-pint) glass of lukewarm water and dispensing it from a spray bottle. You should spray into each nostril while pinching off the other nostril and simultaneously inhaling through your nose. This can be done as often as you'd like throughout the day. It's non-addicting and has no negative side effects that I'm aware of, except for the curious looks you'll get from those wanting to know what in the world you're doing.

A more effective way of moisturizing, but more importantly, irrigating, is saline irrigation. This procedure can result in dramatic relief from pain, since it reduces swelling in the nasal passages, causing a reduction of pressure in the sinus. The salt water sprays that I just mentioned also irrigate, i.e., wash out mucus, bacteria, dust particles, etc., while reducing swelling. But they don't do it as well as the following methods, which should be used three to four times a day.

Make the irrigating (saline) solution fresh each day in one cup of lukewarm tap water. Add ¼ to ½ teaspoon of table salt and a tiny pinch of baking soda, thus making the solution close to normal body fluid salinity and pH. Irrigating with plain water is usually somewhat uncomfortable. Use the full cup of saline solution for each irrigation (one-half cup for each nostril), and irrigate with the head over the sink but in an upright position. Always blow the nose *very* gently after irrigating.

Method 1: Completely fill a large all-rubber ear syringe (available at most pharmacies) with saline solution. Lean over sink and pinch one nostril closed. Insert syringe tip just inside open nostril, pinching nostril around tip. *Gently* squeeze bulb and release several times to swish solution around inside nose. Solution will run out both nostrils and may also run out mouth. Repeat for each nostril until one cup of saline solution is used, or until the solution is clear.

Method 2: Pour saline solution into palm of hand and sniff solution up nose, one nostril at a time.

Method 3: Use angled nasal irrigator attachment (Grossman nasal irrigator, available at some pharmacies) on a Water Pik appliance. Set Water Pik at lowest possible pressure and insert irrigator tip just inside nostril, pinching nostril to seal. Irrigate with mouth open, allowing fluid to drain out either mouth or nose.

Method 4: For very small children, irrigate with ten to twenty drops of saline solution per nostril from an eyedropper.

If you are using a decongestant nasal spray, use it only AFTER the salt water nasal irrigations.

This method obviously requires more effort than the saline nasal sprays, but many patients have commented on how helpful it has been.

Another solution that has been effective in irrigation is called Alkalol. It is a mucus solvent and cleaner, and can be used with the saline solution in a 1:1 ratio (½ saline, ½ Alkalol) with all of the above methods. You'll probably have to ask your pharmacist to order it for you, as it is not usually available. It's very inexpensive.

HYDRATION AND BED REST

How often have you heard the advice, "Drink lots of liquids and stay in bed"? Even with acute sinusitis it still holds true. I recommend at least eight to ten 8-ounce glasses of water daily. Avoid ice-cold drinks and anything with caffeine, sugar, or alcohol.

As for resting, try to listen to your body and not push yourself. As a general rule, if you are waking up to an alarm clock then you're not getting enough sleep. Allow your body to tell you how much sleep you need and adjust your bedtime accordingly. Do as much resting as possible during the first five to seven days of treatment.

MISCELLANEOUS

Many physicians have their own special sinus remedies in addition to the medically approved regimen that I have just described. Several that are frequently mentioned, but with which I have no personal experience, are a combination of topical caffeine and Ocean spray; Argyrol, a silver solution used as an antiinfective drop in the nose; and Ichthyol 20 percent in glycerin, applied as a nasal packing to open the ostia and sinus ducts and draw infected mucus out of the sinuses.

In many cases, acute sinusitis coexists as a "silent partner" with a more recognizable ailment. The most common instances will be discussed in Chapter 5. Sinus infections in these circumstances should be treated with much the same methods that have been described in this chapter. For additional help in treating acute sinusitis please refer to Chapter 10, with specific regard to diet, vitamins, herbs, and nutritional supplements.

Chapter 5

When Acute Sinusitis Coexists with Other Medical Conditions

It is not uncommon for acute sinusitis to coexist with other conditions that also affect the respiratory tract. In almost every instance when this occurs, it is the accompanying problem, not the sinus infection, that is most apparent to both physician and patient. Two of these problems—the common cold and nasal allergies—precede the onset of acute sinusitis, while the others occur subsequent to the sinus infection.

THE COMMON COLD

This is the most frequent condition concomitant with sinusitis. Since it has been discussed from different perspectives in Chapters 2, 3, and 4, there is little left to say. I will, however, remind you that if you're at all suspicious of a sinus infection, or you're at high risk for getting one, then avoid taking antihistamines. Every cold can be treated in the same way that I recommended for acute sinusitis, with the exception of the antibiotic. If the sinus infection is present along with the cold, it should become obvious in seven to ten days.

ACUTE OTITIS MEDIA (MIDDLE EAR INFECTION)

This is quite commonly seen in children, and very often in conjunction with acute sinusitis. The bacteria that cause this infection are identical to those responsible for sinus infections. The position and anatomy of the eustachian tube, which drains the middle ear space, helps to create the simultaneous infections. I once heard an ENT physician say that any time you see an adult with otitis media, that person always has an under-lying acute sinusitis.

When otitis media is present, sinusitis is usually ignored or not even recognized. Most of these patients are extremely un-comfortable with ear pain, and that becomes the focus of attention for both doctor and patient. Young children will also usually have a significant (above 101° F) fever. The treatment of otitis media can be exactly the same as that of acute sinusitis, so that even if the diagnosis of sinusitis is missed, the sinus in-fection usually will get better anyway. In adults with otitis media, however, I would recommend more regular use of a de-congestant than I would for children, and for a longer period of time than I would with sinusitis (three times a day for at least ten days). This is because adults with middle ear infections routinely complain of "stuffiness" in their ears long after the pain has gone, often for two to three weeks.

Many young children have repeated episodes of acute otitis media, as often as four or five times within a year. Family physicians and pediatricians are very familiar with this kind of patient. What is probably happening with most of them is that each cold they get quickly becomes a sinus infection, which then causes the ear infection. Since the average number of colds per year in young kids can be as great as six, that can oc-casion lots of visits to the doctor or an emergency room (ear in-fections often begin at night). Many of these pediatric patients will eventually require surgery (involving the placement of tubes through the eardrums).

ALLERGIC RHINITIS (NASAL ALLERGY)

When allergies accompany sinusitis, or the patient suffering from allergy symptoms is known to have a history of sinus in-fections, the problem becomes one of the more challenging ones in medicine. Since allergy results in swelling and inflam-mation of the nasal mucous membrane and blockage of the sinus ducts, it is important to be able to treat these symptoms without creating a sinus infection. An acute flare-up of a runny nose and cough or difficulty controlling nasal congestion with the usual allergy therapy may signal the presence of a sinus in-fection.

Most people with seasonal nasal allergy, also known as hay fever, rely upon over-the-counter medications for relief. Many of these I mentioned in Chapter 4, e.g., Dristan, Contac, Allerest, Drixoral, Actifed, Dimetapp, Triaminicin, and Sudafed-Plus. They are helpful primarily because of the anti-histamine that they all contain in addition to a decongestant. Chlortrimeton is another popular one, but without a decongestant. Antihistamines are wonderful drugs for the treatment of allergies, although they do cause drowsiness. Seldane and Hismanal, two of the latest prescription antihistamines, are very popular exceptions. Not only are they not sedating, but they also seem to cause much less thickening of the mucus. For this reason, I would recommend them for allergy sufferers who are also prone to developing sinus infections. If you have allergies in conjunction with weak sinuses or a current sinus infection, please avoid the OTC antihistamines.

Another option for treating nasal allergies in a sinus sufferer is to use Nasalcrom, Beconase, and Vancenase sprays. All are prescription drugs. Nasalcrom is a topical mast-cell inhibitor, which simply means that it prevents an allergic reaction from taking place on the nasal mucous membrane but is not absorbed into the body. Beconase and Vancenase are cortisone nasal sprays that act similarly. They have both an antiallergic and antiinflammatory effect. These nasal sprays work even better if used after nasal irrigation (described in the "Moisture and Irrigation" section of Chapter 4). Irrigation will remove the mucus secretions so the prescription spray won't sit on the mucus, but will directly hit the lining of the nose. The irrigation will remove allergens (pollen) as well.

In the case of a seasonal allergy sufferer, the spray should be used throughout the season. The majority of people with hay fever are reacting either to tree pollen (April-May), grasses (May-June), or weeds (August-September). The seasonal use of the spray applies to all those with allergy symptoms having a history of sinus infections. They'll not only obtain effective relief for their symptoms, but likely will also avoid both the acute sinusitis and the drowsiness potentially caused by OTC antihistamines. Treatment with prescription nasal sprays is not, however, without its long-term side effects. Long-term use of the cortisone sprays can cause chronic irritation, inflammation, and increased mucus secretion. I've seen several patients develop terrible coughs resulting from severe postnasal drip after using the sprays for several months. In the humid southern states, molds can be a significant problem all year long. In these situations I'd recommend using the sprays only during the most severe periods of allergic reaction—probably not year-round, because of the side effects I've just described. Chapters 8 and 10 contain information that should help in coping with continuous allergies.

If someone already has an acute sinusitis along with the hay fever, which can be a very difficult diagnosis to make, the patient should use the regular sinusitis treatment regimen in addition to Nasalcrom, the cortisone sprays, Seldane, or Hismanal. Some of these people are so uncomfortable that I'll add a short course of cortisone tablets.

BRONCHITIS AND PNEUMONIA

I've already described in Chapter 3 the condition called sinobronchitis, i.e., sinusitis coexisting with bronchitis. It is being seen with greater frequency and is also not a simple diagnosis to make. The cough is usually the primary complaint. It is a persistent (day and night), deep, wet, and mucusy (yellow) cough, often found in smokers. The usual symptoms of sinusitis are also present. Needless to say, these people seem more ill than the typical acute sinusitis patient.

Worse yet are those whose bronchitis has turned into pneumonia, which is simply a more severe lung infection than the bronchitis. These patients are quite sick with a bad cough and often fever and chills.

Both of these lung infections can usually be diagnosed by listening to the lungs with a stethoscope; pneumonia can be confirmed with a chest X-ray. When a sinus infection is also present, it most likely will have preceded these lung conditions and probably created them with the postnasal drainage of infected mucus into the lungs.

Following the diagnosis, the next step lies in selecting an antibiotic that will cure both infections. It will be difficult to get rid of the infection in the lungs if the sinusitis is still present. It is for this reason that I will not choose erythromycin to start treatment. Although it may be the best choice for the lungs, I have seen many instances in which it was ineffective in treating a sinus infection. Several of the broad-spectrum antibiotics listed in Table 1 would be a good choice. The rest of the treatment program is the same as it is for sinusitis, with the addition of postural drainage techniques to help clear the lungs of infection.

ASTHMA

This is another disease of the lungs that is very much affected by sinusitis. In a study published in 1987 by the National Jewish Center for Immunology and Respiratory Medicine in Denver, a national research center for asthma and other respiratory diseases, it was noted that more than two-thirds of the patients in the study with mild to severe asthma had sinus abnormalities on X-ray. It was also reported that sinus treatment of asthmatic children with moderate to severe sinus abnormalities may improve their asthma. The study made reference to a report completed in 1925 that postulated four mechanisms that might explain how sinus disease could cause asthma. Those conclusions were not substantially different from the ones made in the 1987 study. Two of these mechanisms are quite similar to what was mentioned in Chapter 3 with respect to the symptoms of cough, sore throat, and laryngitis. They are (1) postnasal drip of mucus into the lower airways, which either directly alters the airways' reactivity or causes the airways' inflammation, and (2) mouth breathing of cold and/or dry air due to nasal obstruction, which elicits asthma by increasing heat and water loss in the lower airways.

The National Jewish Center treats primarily asthmatics who are poorly controlled and/or steroid (cortisone) dependent. (Ironically, the hospital sits in one of the highest air pollution locations in the entire city. In a national survey released in September 1989, doctors reported seeing a dramatic increase in asthma patients. The reason most frequently cited by the physicians for the growing number of patients is air pollution.) The center's study linking sinus disease to asthma described many asthmatics who improved dramatically and were able to decrease their steroid requirements following treatment of their sinusitis. If this holds true for the worst asthmatics, then it should also apply to anyone with mild to moderate asthma who is experiencing a flare-up or an exacerbation of their condition. If an obvious cause for the asthmatic episode is not present, e.g., common cold, allergy, exercise, emotional stress, etc., and the wheezing can't be controlled with the usual medication, then think of the possibility of a sinus infection.

That is also the message for the other conditions described in this chapter. I am trying to instill a greater level of awareness of the existence of sinusitis. Not only can the sinus infection be subtle in its presentation, but when it accompanies these other conditions, it can have a profound impact on the course of the illness.

Most people suffering from a sinus infection will find the treatment program described in Chapter 4 quite effective both in relieving their discomfort and in eliminating the infection. However, for the growing number of people who have had repeated episodes of acute sinusitis and are now chronic sinus sufferers; for those who are seeking an alternative to the traditional medical approach; and for anyone interested in preventive medicine and in understanding how lifestyle contributes to the cause of sinus disease, Part II will be your next step to better health.

Part II

Treating Chronic Sinusitis:
An Approach to Holistic Health

Chapter 6

Traditional Medicine

The treatment for chronic sinusitis consists primarily of antibiotics and surgery. These are traditional medicine's biggest guns, and although they are assisted by decongestants, expectorants, antitussives, analgesics, moisture, irrigation (see Chapter 4), and cortisone nasal sprays, antibiotics and surgery remain the foundation for treating America's most common chronic disease. Obviously if this approach had a high rate of success, i.e., a high cure rate, we would probably not be experiencing an epidemic in which nearly one out of every seven Americans suffers from a chronic sinus condition.

Although medical science continues to create stronger antibiotics and develop more effective surgical techniques, we seem to be winning battles but losing the war against sinus disease. Otolaryngologists (ear, nose, and throat specialists) are the surgical professionals usually assigned the task of treating the most challenging chronic sinus sufferers—the first group of people I described in Chapter 3 with chronic sinusitis. The people in this group are the most uncomfortable sinus patients. Before arriving at the ENT's office, they have often been fighting a sinus infection for several months to a year, and in many cases, two or three years. Their physicians have given up and consider these patients to be treatment failures. Most of these people have already been through several courses of antibiotics without success.

The initial evaluation by the ENT doctor usually includes a physical examination of the nose, throat, and sinuses following the application of a topical decongestant in the nose, and a nasal bacterial culture as well. The specimen for this culture needs to be obtained right from the opening of the sinus ducts (ostia) or else it will be of little value. In his evaluation the ENT physician is attempting to identify the specific bacteria that are infecting the sinuses. The bacteria found in the nose are not usually the same as those that are infecting the sinuses. Therefore, it is important that the culture be performed by someone who has had a lot of experience in locating the ostia (usually an ENT physician), so that the results will be a true reflection of the bacteria that are actually causing the infection. This test is critical for the selection of the best antibiotic. Many specialists have seen a dramatic increase in the prevalence of *Staphylococcus aureus* in the sinuses as a result of the more accurate performance of this test. Not surprisingly, this is one of the most difficult bacteria to treat.

Subsequent diagnostic procedures might include a sinus CT scan to determine if, after a course of an antibiotic, there are any lingering pockets of infection; rhinoscopy—the insertion of a flexible "telescope" into the nasal passages to see if there is any obstruction around the ostia (this procedure is probably performed more often by allergists than by ENT physicians); a nasal cytogram—a microscopic inspection of cells from the nasal mucous membrane; and a complete battery of skin and/or blood tests to identify possible allergies. For additional information on the diagnosis of chronic sinusitis, refer to Chapter 3.

The initial treatment usually includes a ten-day to two-week course of one of the strongest antibiotics—Cipro, Ceftin, or Suprax (not effective for *Staphylococcus*)—in addition to the treatment regimen described in Chapter 4, with particular emphasis on irrigation. If this fails—either there is no improvement, or infection is still present on the CT scan, or the infection recurs shortly after the antibiotic is stopped—then further evaluation will be necessary using one or more of the diagnostic procedures just mentioned. Depending upon the results, either another antibiotic or surgery will be offered as the next step.

Sinus surgery has improved dramatically in the past three years. If there is obstruction of the ostio-meatal complex (the opening of the sinus duct into the nasal passage), surgery is usually recommended. The endoscope, another type of flexible "telescope," has taken sinus surgery to another level of success. The most common endoscopic surgical procedure is a bilateral middle antrostomy, in which the maxillary sinus ostia are enlarged from 2 millimeters to about 10 or 12 millimeters (approximately the size of a dime). This is a marked improvement from the naso-antral windows that used to be created surgically. The opening of a naso-antral window was about the same size as the opening created by an antrostomy, but it went entirely through the bony medial wall (nasal side) of the maxillary sinus. The new procedure is not only less destructive, but more importantly, it preserves the normal direction of mucus flow in the sinus. Mucus naturally flows out through the sinus duct and into the nose. The fact that the naso-antral window was not in the best position to enhance drainage greatly diminished its rate of success, despite the large opening it produced. Many patients who have had this surgery as well as the Caldwell-Luc operation and ethmoidectomy (other common surgical procedures not often performed anymore) continue to have sinus problems and not infrequently have had additional surgery. Endoscopic surgery so far looks very good. It is performed on an outpatient basis under local anesthesia, and patients can expect to miss about one week of work. It is certainly not inexpensive—surgeons will charge anywhere from $4000 to $10,000 to do the procedure. Following the surgery, patients are often instructed to use Nasalcrom or one of the cortisone sprays for several months. Since it has been popular for only about three years, long-term success rates for endoscopic surgery are not yet available. However, it is clearly an improvement over the previous procedures.

Sinus surgery has been and will probably continue to be most successful in those instances when it is being performed to eliminate one of the obstructive causes of sinusitis, e.g., a deviated septum, an enlarged or distorted nasal turbinate (turbinate hypertrophy), cysts, or polyps. In these cases the surgery eliminates causes, but where there is no obstruction the surgery will only be treating symptoms, and whatever the underlying factors that created the chronic sinusitis, they will still be present following surgery. This is precisely why chronic sinusitis is usually considered to be an incurable condition. Whether the chronic sinus sufferer has repeated debilitating infections over several years; a more mild subtle infection with fatigue over most of a lifetime; or a persistent inflammation resulting in congestion, headaches, postnasal drip, and a weakened sense of smell and taste, the traditional medical approach for the most part offers symptomatic treatment along with the prognosis, "You're going to have to learn to live with it."

Chapter 7

Holistic Medicine: Introduction

If you would rather not "learn to live with it," accepting the fate of a diminished quality of life, but would prefer to "smell the roses," then I'd like to take you on a journey into an exciting new frontier of medicine. This option for treating chronic sinusitis is one I have been using for the past four years. Whenever someone has made a commitment to try this approach, it has resulted in a 100 percent success rate in either significantly improving or curing the condition. It is *not* an alternative to traditional medicine but a complement. In confronting an incurable disease, why not choose a treatment program that incorporates many therapeutic modalities, not merely those that have been officially sanctioned by medical science? I strongly believe that everything mentioned in the remainder of this chapter will eventually be validated by the scientific community (much of it already has been). Until that occurs, I will persist in attesting to the remarkable efficacy of this method while continuing to refine it.

Holistic medicine is a unique blend of health education and medical treatment. Health is regarded as a state of wholeness (the word "health" comes from the Anglo-Saxon word "haelen," meaning "to make whole") and balance, and as a result of practicing holistic medicine an individual will experience a heightened sense of physical, mental, emotional, spiritual, and social well-being. Holistic medicine encompasses elements of allopathic (whose practitioners are M.D.s), osteopathic (D.O.s), chiropractic (D.C.s), naturopathic (N.D.s), Chinese (O.M.D.s), environmental, and preventive medicine and is based in part upon the science of psychoneuroimmunology. The doctor ("doctor" is a Latin word meaning "teacher") works in partnership with patients to guide them through their own process of self-healing. Rather than being a fixer of the "broken" part of the body, a holistic physician becomes a teacher of health, enabling patients to take better care of their body, mind, emotions, spirit, and relationships. The admonition of the physician-philosopher Hippocrates, "Physician, heal thyself," is still being taught to medical students, 2400 years after the words were first spoken. It is an invitation to the physician to discover the power of the healing process in the only way it can be discovered—through personal experience. Hippocrates was saying that if physicians are health educators, the best way to teach is to practice what you preach.

This approach is directed toward treating causes rather than symptoms and unfortunately does not often lend itself to the "quick fix" to which we have become so accustomed in our society. Whether our need is food, energy, entertainment, transportation, communication, or health care, we continue to look for the fast, simple, and easy solutions. Science and technology have attempted to keep pace with those desires, and indeed, they have performed incredible, at times almost miraculous feats that have allowed an ease of living never before experienced in human history. However, there is a price to be paid. Technology is helping us to rapidly destroy our environment—polluting our air, poisoning our food and water, depleting our soil, thinning our protective ozone layer, decimating our forests at the rate of one acre every second, and causing the extinction of nearly one hundred species of plants and animals daily! Our own species, *Homo sapiens*, may not be far behind.

Sinus disease is the first environmental epidemic to affect mankind. There is already evidence to indicate that it may soon be followed by lung disease and all types of cancer, especially skin cancer. Lung cancer has shown the greatest increase of any form of cancer in the United States in the past forty years. Asthma, the most common chronic childhood disease, is attacking and killing more young children now than it did twenty years ago. Emphysema, too, is increasing. Physicians are beginning to recognize the magnitude of the health hazards of air pollution.

In order to treat these conditions most effectively, a twofold external/internal approach is necessary. This entails minimizing and if possible eliminating the harmful environmental factors that have contributed to causing the condition (external), in addition to strengthening the body itself and its natural defense mechanism, the immune system (internal). Chapter 8 will focus on external treatment, and Chapters 9 through 14 will explore the various aspects of internal treatment.

Chapter 8

External Treatment: Environmental Medicine

There is nothing more important to human health than the quality of the air we breathe. Oxygen is the single factor most critical to human survival. We can survive without eating for about a month, without water for several days, but without air death is only minutes away. The sinuses, our first line of defense against unhealthy air, can become a sensitive gauge (especially in sinus sufferers) to determine air quality. There are five aspects of optimum air: clarity (air that is free of pollutants), humidity (between 40 and 60 percent), temperature (between 65° and 85° F), oxygen content (21 percent of total volume and 100 percent saturation), and negative ion content (3000 to 6000 .001-micron ions per cubic centimeter). Air that is clean, moist, warm, oxygen rich, and high in negative ions is the healthiest air a human being can breathe. Pollution, humidity, and temperature have all been discussed in Chapter 2. Not only are we dependent on oxygen for our survival, but every part of the human body thrives with a maximum supply of oxygen. If your respiratory tract is defective because of a nasal, sinus, or lung ailment, or if the amount of oxygen available in the air is relatively low (e.g., air high in carbon monoxide, air at higher altitudes, or stale indoor air), then your body is receiving less than its optimal requirement of oxygen.

Negative ions are electrically charged particles that vitalize or freshen the air. Studies have shown that they can help to create a feeling of well-being while reducing pain, healing burns, suppressing bacterial growth, stimulating plant growth, and improving the sweeping motion of the cilia on the mucous membrane. The highest concentrations of negative ions have been found on mountaintops, along seacoasts, by rushing streams and waterfalls, and in pine forests (pine needles and the pointed leaves of other plants give off negative ions through the points). Most people who have spent time in these environments have described feeling very good or at least experiencing an improvement in their sense of well-being, and although there are certainly other factors involved, negative ions are a significant contributor to the experience.

The majority of Americans spend 90 percent of their time indoors, where, the EPA says, the air can be as much as 100 times more polluted than outdoor air. In Chapter 2 I've listed most of the more common indoor air pollutants. Most of us do not live in clean, moist, and warm year-round environments and also do not live in the mountains, on a beach, or in the woods. For the 34 million people whose sinuses are already feeling the pain created by breathing unhealthy air, and for anyone else who would like to enjoy optimum health, what can be done to minimize the health risks of breathing poor-quality indoor air as well as to prevent sinus disease?

LOCATION

Where we live, work, play, or otherwise spend our time is critical to indoor air quality and our health. If you are considering a move, the following list of factors will help in evaluating a location.

— Locate homes and buildings to minimize the impact of outdoor air pollution.
— Locate in a city, town, or county that has minimal air pollution.
— Locate on a hill rather than a valley where pollution is more apt to concentrate.
— Do not locate near a major highway or traffic intersection.
— Do not locate next to a parking lot.
— Do not locate downwind from a power plant, chemical plant, or processing plant.
— Do not locate near industrial operations.
— Do not locate near local businesses that exhaust pollutants.

— Do not locate near a railroad line that carries hazardous materials.
— Do not locate near airfields.
— Do not locate on land farmed with pesticides and chemical fertilizers.
— Locate away from agricultural fields that are sprayed.
— Do not live under or near high-voltage power lines.
— Locate away from stagnant waterways.
— Locate out of air pollution or "seepage" range of oil or gas wells.
— Locate a safe distance from any mining operations.
— Locate close to a park, near a forest, or within a natural setting.
— Locate in a small healthful rural or seacoast community.
— Consider the effect of altitude on air quality.
— Consider prevailing diurnal and seasonal wind patterns.
— Before moving to a city, review an air quality record of the past several years.
— In urban or rural locations, consider sites for passive solar orientation and exposure.
— South-sloping sites are preferable for drainage and solar advantage.
— Avoid being in a "shadow path" during winter months in a cold climate.
— Avoid sites with high levels of radon or radioactivity.
— Before buying a property, get soils, radon, and water tests (if a well is planned).
— Check municipal water quality.*

It is unlikely that all of these locational criteria can be met, but they can provide a basis for a thorough evaluation. If you are going to relocate and have the freedom to choose anyplace in the United States, I would avoid the following regions: Southern California, the Northeast, and the Texas Gulf Coast; the following states: Ohio, Texas, Illinois, Michigan, Indiana, New Jersey, Connecticut, and Tennessee; and the following

---

* Reprinted with permission from *Indoor Air: Risks and Remedies,* by Richard L. Crowther.

cities: Los Angeles, New York, Chicago, Philadelphia, St. Louis, Houston, Denver, Memphis, and Las Vegas. The healthiest air can be found along the West Coast (with the distinct exception of the L.A. metropolitan area and southward) and anywhere in Hawaii other than Honolulu.

ECOLOGICAL ARCHITECTURE

If you are contemplating the construction of a new home, the concepts of ecological architecture could help considerably in creating a healthy environment. Ecology is defined in Webster's *New World Dictionary* as "the branch of biology that deals with the relationship between living organisms and their environment." In this instance it simply means the design of a dwelling that is sensitive to human health and gentle to the earth. Nature, with respect to the microclimate and the site, dictates the design in accordance with our biologic needs, behavior patterns, and, most importantly, our budgetary limitations. Self-sufficiency by using sun, air, earth, and water for heating, cooling, ventilation, and solar-powered electricity is a realistic goal of an ecological design.

Common objectives regarding construction methods and materials include:

— to avoid plastic or other materials made of toxic ingredients that harmfully outgas in the indoor environment;
— use of nontoxic natural materials in preference to synthetic materials;
— design concern for sensitivities, allergies, or chronic health problems;
— concern that Nature's ecologic sustainability and well-being should not be diminished by what is built; and
— a responsibility to conceive, design, build, and furnish a home or building to a "healthy home" ecologic ethic.*

This is a holistic approach encompassing health, vitality, and viability in the ecological bond between site and architecture.

* Reprinted with permission from *Indoor Air: Risks and Remedies,* by Richard L. Crowther.

To preserve and wisely use our planet's resources initially in construction and through the lifetime of the home is fundamental to ecological design. For the sinus sufferer a home must be clean, moist, warm, and oxygen and negative ion rich as well as extremely energy efficient. The fact that it is designed in harmony with the atmosphere and the earth makes this a totally integrated concept.

I fully appreciate that most readers of this book will neither move nor design their own home. However, I want to present as many environmental treatment options as possible. Each of them is capable of having a profound impact on your state of health and ultimately your quality of life.

HEALTHY HOMES

Since most of you will not be moving to Hawaii (that's good, because if everybody did, there would be one less place to which we could escape for a vacation), I have attempted to create the next best thing—an oasis of healthy indoor air in your own home. In the desert an oasis provides water. In the "sea" of hazardous air in which we live, a healthy home or business can provide an air oasis in which to breathe life-enhancing vitalized air.

Over the past two years I have met with air filtration, humidification, negative ionization, and indoor air pollution experts; allergists; specialists in environmental medicine; ecological architects; and energy-efficient builders. With their guidance and the use of state-of-the-art technology, I am developing an environmental health company called Sinus Survival Products. Born out of the frustration of having to send my sinus patients back into the environment that helped to create their ailment in the first place, the company's initial focus is on air treatment. It provides clean, moist, oxygen- and negative ion–rich air. To my knowledge, it is the only company of its kind.

Solving the problem of indoor air pollution entails both treatment and prevention. Treatment involves accepting pollutants (see Chapter 2, "Air Pollution—Indoor") as inevitable components of indoor air and attempting to reduce them as much as possible with air cleaners, negative ion generators, ventilation, and air duct cleaning. Prevention is an attempt to eliminate the sources of the pollutants, especially those you have identified as ones to which you may be most sensitive.

AIR CLEANERS AND
NEGATIVE ION GENERATORS

As many as one million hospital visits per year are now being attributed to poor indoor air quality. In recent years, as the EPA has more fully recognized this problem of indoor air pollution, we have seen a proliferation in this country of several hundred types of air cleaners, almost as many as there are indoor air pollutants. According to Dr. Michael Berry, manager of the EPA's Indoor Air Project, the most potentially harmful pollutants are radon and the "biologicals," i.e., pollen, mold, plant spores, dust mites, bacteria, and viruses. Regardless of their origin, size, or health-damaging effects, air pollutants can basically be described as free-floating particles in the air. Figure E shows the specific size ranges of the most common pollutants. The unit of measurement used for tiny air particles is the micron. An average hair strand is 100 microns thick, and about 400 1-micron particles would fit into the dot over the "i" in the word "micron." The primary job of air cleaners is to remove as many of these particles as possible, the biologicals as well as the combustion products, particulates, chemicals, fumes, and odors—see Table 1. (The amounts of radon, if it is present, are lessened by sealing basement cracks and improving basement ventilation. Air cleaners do not remove radon from the air.)

The strategy for solving the problem of indoor air pollution involves air cleaning and improved ventilation. Sinus Survival Products offers four air cleaners to fit most budgets and home designs. The first three can be attached to a furnace (forced-hot-air type) and clean the air in the entire house, while the fourth is a portable stand-alone unit effective in a bedroom or any single large room. The efficiency of air cleaners is evaluated by their ability to filter a certain percentage of a particular size of pollutant. Sinus Survival–35 is a furnace filter that is over 35 percent effective in removing all particles 1 micron (1/25,000 inch) or larger, and 100 percent effective on particles

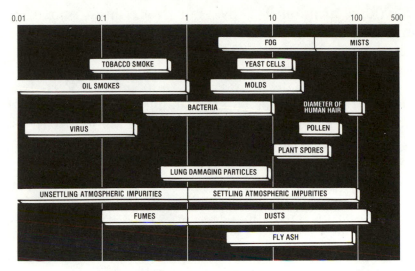

*Figure E. Relative Size of Common
Air Contaminants in Microns.*

5 microns and larger (see Figure E). This includes all pollen, plant spores, most animal dander, the largest particles in household dust, and over 50 percent of all molds and bacteria. It is much more efficient than the commercially available furnace filters found in hardware stores and supermarkets. It can be replaced every three to four months and costs $5.

Sinus Survival–85 is the next step up from the 35, with an 85 percent efficiency on all 1-micron particles and larger. This means that it removes about 70 percent of all the lung-damaging particles that normally go through a standard home furnace filter. These include dust, wood and tobacco smoke (larger particles), fumes, particulates of outdoor pollution, bacteria, and some viruses. Filters of this type are found in most hospital heating and air conditioning systems throughout the United States. The system is designed to be attached to the existing return duct located next to the furnace. This system costs from $350 to $400 depending upon installation costs. Replacement of the $75 filter element is on an annual basis.

Sinus Survival–95 Hepa is a system identical to the 85 except that the 85 percent filter has been replaced with a 95 percent hepa (stands for **h**igh **e**fficiency **p**articulate **a**rrestor) filter. It removes 95 percent of all 0.3-micron particles and larger (everything mentioned above but more dust, smoke, and fumes), and this type is standard equipment for most hospital operating suites. Like the 85, it is designed to attach to the furnace's return duct, except that a booster fan is needed to help move the air through the filter due to its increased efficiency. This system costs about $600 including installation, with replacement of the $130 filter element on an annual basis.

The Sinus Survival Room Unit is a portable stand-alone version of the Sinus Survival–95 Hepa for homes that do not have a central heating system, offices, and any enclosed environment not exceeding 500 square feet (most bedrooms are within this size). Since the majority of American families now have both husband and wife working outside the home, the bulk of the time spent at home is in the bedroom. This system needs only to be plugged into a 110-volt outlet. It costs $450 and the $130 filter element requires annual replacement.

The Sinus Survival–85, –95, and Room Unit can all be equipped with odor- and gas-filtering systems. An add-on negative ionization system for the Room Unit is currently under development. In addition to vitalizing the air, negative ions have the capacity to remove particles as small as .001 micron. This would include all viruses, dust, and all outdoor air pollutants. Negative ion generator units are presently available in a variety of shapes, sizes, and prices. Their primary liability is that since the negatively charged particles are free in the air, they will attach to the nearest grounding surface. This means that dirty residues will accumulate on metal objects, including unseen nails used for drywall. This problem can be minimized by placing the ionizer at least two feet away from any wall or ceiling surface and using a strategically located positive magnetic field plate to attract the dirt-laden ionized particles.

Electrostatic air cleaners (both central and free standing) produce negative ions as they filter the air. On their first day of operation they are as efficient as the Sinus Survival–85, but in order to maintain that efficiency they require cleaning every two weeks. For most of us, this makes them impractical and inconvenient. They also produce ozone, which, as I've already discussed in Chapter 2, can be a potential health hazard.

AIR DUCT CLEANING

Recently I learned of a service I never knew existed. A Denver company called Monster Vac thoroughly cleaned the entire air duct system in my home for the first time. I was amazed by what emanated from the air ducts of my thirteen-year-old home after two hours of high-intensity vacuuming. I thought to myself, "It's no wonder I suffered with sinus problems for so long!" It is nearly impossible to adequately clean the air in your home with a furnace filter, no matter how effective it may be, if the air ducts are filthy. After the air is filtered it still has to travel through the ducts before you breathe it. I highly recommend air duct cleaning as part of the environmental treatment program. Depending upon the size of your home, the cost could be between $200 and $250. To find this type of company in your city, look in the yellow pages of the phone book under "Furnaces, Cleaning and Repairing."

VENTILATION, OXYGEN, AND PLANTS

All indoor spaces, whether residential, commercial/industrial, or recreational, require ventilation to provide breathable air for the occupants, to furnish combustion air for cooking and heating, and to remove stale air filled with toxins and particulates. Commercial buildings are required by code to have ventilation. Ventilation standards of the American Society of Heating, Refrigerating and Air-Conditioning Engineers (ASHRAE) require that air be replaced at the rate of 15 cubic feet per minute per person, but most buildings are unable to comply with this requirement.

Improving and increasing ventilation will help relieve indoor air pollution as long as the outdoor air isn't more polluted than what it's replacing inside. Local pollution sources, such as fumes from toxic waste leakage, wood burning in fireplaces, a neighboring industrial plant, a heavily trafficked highway, or crop spraying can render outdoor air unacceptable for indoor ventilation. For a total of almost two weeks out of every year, Los Angeles residents are advised to keep all windows and doors closed and ventilation ducts shut to prevent the heavily polluted outdoor air from entering homes and businesses. In areas like this, it becomes a challenge to balance the health (survival) benefits of obtaining oxygenated outdoor air with the liability of all the pollutants that accompany the oxygen. Doing outdoor aerobic exercise presents a similar dilemma. If you live in a heavily polluted environment, I would recommend exercising and ventilating your home and office well when outdoor air is good, and keeping windows and doors closed during periods of heavy pollution.

Air-conditioning systems are a helpful means of ventilation for people with respiratory and allergy problems. These systems cool by removing moisture from the air and by lowering its temperature. In less humid conditions there is a reduction of molds and spores, and with the windows closed there is also a marked decrease in pollen from the outdoors.

Natural cross-ventilation is effective in reducing indoor air pollution if the placement of the intake vents is low and the outlets for the flow-through air are high. Operable windows on commercial buildings and a good location for the outdoor air intake (e.g., not near a garage entrance or a loading dock) are also important factors in improving indoor air quality. Mechanical ventilation with exhaust fans can certainly help in removing indoor pollutants, but such fans are most efficient when used in a confined space. For instance, private offices or single-occupant rooms where smoking, cooking, and other fume-producing activities occur are ideal environments for mechanical ventilation.

Rooms producing commercial toxic or odoriferous fumes, spaces subject to bacterial and viral contamination (e.g., restrooms), and other indoor areas that present specific respiratory hazards need optimized ventilation. Mold especially is quite prolific in moist conditions. Adequate ventilation along with sunshine can help to reduce moisture and subsequently suppress mold.

The technology of ventilation can be complex, but the basic principle of displacing interior air with outdoor air and increasing the rate of fresh air flow is critical to treating the problem of indoor air pollution. Besides natural cross-ventilation and exhaust fans, other devices used to enhance ventilation and indoor air quality are air-to-air heat exchangers, make-up air units, attic fans, vortex fans, and ceiling fans. Remember that even if the "fresh" air is filthy, an effective air cleaner combined with good ventilation is still a winning combination.

Along with ventilation upgrading, sealing a building's exterior may prove to be the least costly as well as the most effective means of improving indoor air quality. Mountain Dwellings, a home construction company in Evergreen, Colorado, does just that. To my knowledge, they build the healthiest and most energy-efficient homes in Colorado. They construct airtight homes with almost no leakage, and continuously fresh indoor air is provided through whole-house controlled ventilation. Heating bills are typically less than $100 per year for a 2500-square-foot home with natural gas or propane as a fuel. (Most of these homes have been built above a 7000-foot elevation, so nights are chilly year-round.)

Adequate ventilation not only helps in reducing indoor air pollution but is the primary source of indoor oxygen. Plants can offer an esthetically pleasant complement in both of these areas. Although the oxygen output from indoor plants is not great, plants with large leaf surfaces that grow rapidly are capable of enhancing air quality. Attached greenhouses and atria filled with plants that effectively absorb carbon dioxide and oxygenate the air (spider plants do this very well) can add a great deal to the indoor environment in addition to humidifying the air.

In recent years, studies conducted at the John Stennis Space Center in Mississippi have shown that plants can also act as effective filters. Researchers estimate that in the average home, fifteen spider plants could remove the formaldehyde emissions from furniture, walls, and cooking. Aloe vera and philodendren plants were also found to reduce levels of formaldehyde, benzene, and carbon dioxide.

I have already mentioned that pine needles and the leaves of other pointed-leaf plants (primarily evergreens) give off negative ions through the points. It's probably unlikely that you'd have room for an evergreen in your living room—though you might fit in a Norfolk Island pine. But the most important point to note is how valuable an asset plants can be to improving indoor air, as oxygenators, filters, humidifiers, and negative ion generators.

PREVENTION

Prevention of indoor air pollution involves eliminating pollutants at the source, especially those you can identify as the ones to which you are most sensitive. Doctors who specialize in environmental medicine can do skin and blood tests to help with the identification process. These doctors are not always easy to find, nor are the tests always definitive, but they can help. Through the use of ecological architectural principles, the ultimate healthy home can be created. A major preventive strategy is the use of materials in indoor environments that emit no pollutants. Natural materials, e.g., wood, cotton, and metals, are preferable to the lower-cost synthetic materials such as fiberboard, polyester, and plastics.

Choosing to forgo a fireplace or wood-burning stove would be helpful, as would using a high-efficiency furnace with a sealed combustion unit to vent exhaust gases to the outside. Switch to nontoxic cleaning substances, e.g., ordinary soap, vinegar, zephiran, Air Therapy (you can find a listing of such cleaners in *Nontoxic, Natural, and Earthwise*, by Debra Dadd). Smoking should be relegated to the outdoors or to a well-ventilated enclosed space. If radon levels exceed the acceptable ASHRAE standard, radon control measures should be implemented. Formaldehyde from insulation can be eliminated by using the substitutes of cellulose and fiberglass insulation.

HUMIDIFICATION

Optimum indoor air quality requires air that contains between 40 and 60 percent relative humidity. I have already discussed the benefits for sinus sufferers of moisture provided by room humidifiers in the "Moisture and Irrigation" section in Chapter 4. Even in humid cold-weather climates, these humidifiers are quite helpful in the winter (heavy "sinus season" runs from November through March), since most heating systems dry the indoor air considerably.

Central humidifiers, those that attach to the furnace, are more convenient but do not humidify an individual room as well as an ultrasonic can when the door to the room is closed. The major problem with central humidifiers is that most of them are the reservoir type, with a tray of standing water that breeds mold and bacteria. Sinus Survival Products provides a flow-through type of central humidifier. This type eliminates the stagnant water problem and is easy to maintain. Depending upon the model, size of your home, and installation, this humidifier would probably cost about $300.

Humidifiers are not the only option for moisturizing your home. The installation of waterfalls, indoor spas, and swimming pools will all add lots of moisture to the house, but, of course, they are expensive to install and maintain. Plants are also good moisturizers.

Another exciting benefit of the airtight homes built by Mountain Dwellings is their ability to maintain a humidity level above 40 percent without any special equipment. The moisture from human breath and sweat, along with cooking, baths, showers, and plants, is enough to do the job, even in a climate as dry as Colorado's.

Chapter 9

Introduction to Internal Treatment: The Body and the Immune System

In reconsidering the most common causes of sinus disease, listed in Chapter 2, you can see how the traditional medical approach and environmental treatment are able to either eliminate or minimize the effects of physical malformations, cigarettes, air pollution (both indoor and outdoor), dry air, cold air, allergies, and occupational hazards. In Chapters 9 through 14, I will describe the internal aspect (the body, and specifically the immune system) of the holistic treatment for chronic sinusitis. This method can reduce or resolve the causal factors of the common cold, allergies, dental problems, immunodeficiency, and emotional stress.

The immune system is that wondrous component of the human body that protects us from all disease. It includes the bone marrow, spleen, liver, lymph nodes, and white blood cells. The study of this field, immunology, is still, relatively speaking, in its infancy. Physicians have empirically known for a long time that if an individual has a sufficient amount of air to breathe, eats a well-balanced diet, drinks enough liquids, and gets enough sleep, he or she should be healthy. The fact that so many of us comply with these basic requirements but get sick anyway has prompted medical research to ask the following questions: Is all air healthy, and if not, what are the components of healthy air? What does a well-balanced, healthy diet consist of? What are the best liquids to drink and how much should we drink? How much sleep do we require? and most importantly, What are the other factors that both weaken and strengthen the immune system? The first question, regarding air quality, I have already answered. In the remainder of this text I will attempt to answer the others, as well as to provide a glimpse of the exciting new (about ten years old) science of psychoneuroimmunology (PNI).

Medical science is presently able to cure about 25 percent of all disease. Traditional medicine and medical training are for the most part disease oriented. As I have mentioned, the focus is on fixing the broken or malfunctioning part of the body that the patient complains most about. This approach is extremely effective in treating acute illness and medical and surgical emergencies. Around 75 percent of the time successful medical treatment means that the symptoms are alleviated until the body's natural healing mechanism in conjunction with the immune system can finish the job (e.g., colds, sore throats, most viral infections); the symptoms are relieved and controlled with long-term medication, surgery, diet, and other measures (e.g., chronic sinusitis, arthritis, diabetes, high blood pressure, allergies); the disease is progressive, debilitating, and often terminal, with variable relief of symptoms with drugs and surgery (e.g., many forms of cancer, Parkinson's, Alzheimer's, many other neurologic diseases, and AIDS).

As medicine now begins to shift its focus from a disease- to a health-oriented approach, the opportunities for curing chronic disease have increased tremendously. At the Harvard University School of Medicine in the Department of Behavioral Medicine, Herbert Benson, M.D., heads the Mind/Body Clinic. Through his scientific research on the "relaxation response" (he is the author of a book with that title), he has shown how relaxation techniques can effectively treat high blood pressure, migraine headaches, and many other common and chronic ailments. He has also documented the healing power of prayer. Bernie Siegel, M.D., of the Yale University School of Medicine, the past president of the American Holistic Medical Association (AHMA) and the author of the bestseller *Love, Medicine, and Miracles*, has had extraordinary results in treating his cancer patients with holistic medicine. C. Norman Shealy, M.D., a neurosurgeon and the cofounder and original president of the AHMA, has been seeing remarkable results for more than fifteen years in the treatment of chronic pain. Dean Ornish, M.D., of the University of California at San Francisco School of Medicine, using a holistic approach has been able to *reverse* coronary artery disease (the leading cause of death in the United States) in his patients—something that has never before been demonstrated. He describes this method in the book *Dr. Dean Ornish's Program for Reversing Heart Disease.*

If holistic medicine has been shown to be effective in treating migraine headaches, high blood pressure, chronic pain, cancer, and heart disease, then surely it can also be used for the nation's most common chronic disease, chronic sinusitis. It does in fact work quite well. The following pages give a brief description of my approach to holistic health and the internal treatment of chronic sinusitis. Each component could warrant an entire book, and I have made reference to several relevant works. My next book, entitled *A Steady State: The Art of Feeling Good*, will describe holistic health in much more depth. However, the program I am presenting here is one I have been teaching for the past four years in the treatment of sinus disease and other chronic conditions. Its focus is on learning to experience greater health and well-being in body, mind, emotions, spirit, and relationships. As by-products of this course of study and of treating the whole person, not only will your sinuses feel better but you will feel a greater sense of aliveness, a vitality, and an enjoyment of life that you may never have experienced before.

Beginning this process of learning to become your own healer requires a commitment to yourself, a willingness to change, an open mind, time, effort, and patience. You can choose to do as much or as little as feels comfortable to you. Many of my patients have experienced great relief from their sinus symptoms after working on just the physical component. However, if you are interested in curing sinus disease, then you must go further. Trust your intuition and remember that, as the "physician" directing this program, you are following a prescription without an exact dosage and, therefore, it isn't possible to make mistakes.

Physical fitness is the first of five aspects of holistic health that will be discussed. Unfortunately, none of the others seems to be as simple, easy, or quick to change as the physical. Believe me, I've tried. Yet the cure for chronic sinusitis and any other chronic disease lies in healing not only the physical but also the less tangible parts of ourselves—the mind, emotions, spirit, and relationships. All of these aspects of health lie beyond the scope of our five senses—vision, hearing, smell, taste, and touch.

This nonphysical aspect of my practice is based upon psychoneuroimmunology—"psycho" meaning mind, "neuro" meaning nervous pathways, and "immuno" meaning immune system. This is a scientific basis of holistic medicine. It could also be called the science of "mind/body" medicine or behavioral medicine. Medical research continues to reveal a wealth of evidence confirming the fact that our thoughts, beliefs, attitudes, emotions, and relationships (both with other people and with a higher power) can strengthen or weaken our immune system. This process occurs in the transmission of messenger molecules (neuropeptides) through the nervous system to be received by the immune system. In the practice of mind/body medicine, the "mind" aspect encompasses mental, emotional, spiritual, and social health. The condition referred to as "stress" or "emotional stress" can result from a problem or an imbalance in any or all of these four aspects of health. A critical factor in the cause of chronic sinusitis and all other disease is this hidden, largely unconscious part of ourselves.

As I practice medicine today, I see myself as a teacher. The course of study I'm teaching is holistic health. Many of my student/patients come to "class" monthly for an extended consultation. They come initially for the treatment of a chronic disease or with the desire to experience a greater degree of health. The majority of these students are chronic sinus sufferers.

I have developed a "curriculum" that has been continually evolving over the past four years. It is designed specifically to implement the principles of mind/body medicine and to help others practice holistic medicine on themselves, as I am doing on myself. There is no doubt that each of us has the potential to become our own best healer. In order to assume greater responsibility for our own health, however, we need first to become better educated.

What follows is a set of healthy options from which to choose (there are also many others) in an approach to holistic health and the implementation of psychoneuroimmunology. Using your intuition to refine and personalize this process of self-healing, you will experience a greater degree of physical fitness, vigor and vitality, peace of mind, ability to use your gifts, awareness of and ability to express feelings, and a greater connectedness with others and with a higher power. You will learn to be more conscious of what feels good and what doesn't and to make choices that are life enhancing. You are, in essence, learning to love yourself, and in so doing you will be better able to love others. This is a program based upon the belief that love is the most powerful healer available to us as human beings. Each of us is the best person to be administering that medicine to ourselves. It is an inexpensive drug without unpleasant side effects, and one on which you cannot overdose.

Chapters 10 through 14 provide a prescription for healing the five components of a human being. I have referred to several books for those who would like to explore these areas in more depth. I've tried to simplify each component and have suggested "exercises" to help you find your own path to a greater level of physical, mental, emotional, spiritual, and social fitness. These exercises must be practiced regularly in order to be effective. (However, if a particular exercise does not feel comfortable to you, don't do it). If you're patient—remember, it took years for you to develop your present state of health—I promise you not only that they will all work, but that every one of them will feel good. Keep in mind that although this is a course with lots of "homework," there are no grades, so enjoy yourself!

Chapter 10

Physical Health

After almost twenty years as a physician it has become quite clear to me that life is not much fun for anyone experiencing physical discomfort or disability. In order to begin working on any other aspect of health (e.g., mental, spiritual), it helps to have some degree of physical stability and symptom relief and some improvement in the degree of pain and/or disability. We do, after all, spend almost all of our time in our bodies.

The objective of physical fitness using the holistic approach is to become more aware of and develop greater respect and appreciation for your body. Through this process you will gain much greater sensitivity to your own body and learn how it functions optimally.

SINUS TREATMENT

Since the majority of you have sinus problems, it is important to begin with an aggressive approach to treating your sinusitis. The same holds true if you are dealing with another chronic condition. Make sure that you have consulted with your physician and have made an attempt to treat your ailment with the best methods that traditional medicine has to offer, even if they only provide symptom relief.

For sinus sufferers this would mean using most of what I have already recommended, i.e., antibiotic, decongestant, expectorant, analgesic, irrigation, saline spray, drinking water, air cleaner, humidifier, negative ion generator, air duct cleaning, and plants. All of these therapeutic modalities for the treatment of sinus disease will make a significant improvement in your condition.

Another option that I am using much more often with chronic sinus patients who have tried frequent courses of antibiotics without success is to treat for systemic yeast infections. Repeated antibiotics can make you much more susceptible to yeast. Yeast (*Candida albicans*) is an "opportunistic" fungus (it's always present but doesn't cause infection until the immune system has been adversely affected). Most commonly it causes vaginal infections in women following a course of an antibiotic. Those infections are generally easy to detect, since most women who have them are well aware of it. Yeast infections in general are much more common in women. Both yeast and antibiotics have been shown to depress immune function, thereby contributing to the cause of chronic sinus infections. There also now seems to be a growing awareness within the medical community that yeast infections are much more prevalent than was previously assumed. An excellent book on this subject is *The Yeast Connection: A Medical Breakthrough,* by William G. Crook, M.D.

Since systemic (whole-body) yeast infections are not easily detected, if the more common antibiotics (see Table 1), are not quite doing the job for your sinus infection, you might want to suggest to your doctor trying a course of Nizoral, a prescription antiyeast antibiotic. It should be taken daily for one month and then every third day for the next month. Neither Nystatin, a prescription drug, nor Cantrol, an over-the-counter alternative that can be found in most health food stores, is as effective as Nizoral. A low-carbohydrate diet can be useful in combatting yeast infections. The degree to which you limit carbohydrates depends upon the severity of the infection. The primary substances to be avoided if yeast is suspected are sugar and yeast. Specifically, eliminate fruits and fruit juices, breads, grains, potatoes, fermented foods (i.e., all alcohol products, cheeses, and pickled foods), leavened and baked goods, mushrooms, and vitamins made with a yeast base. This is a diet consisting primarily of vegetables and protein.

DIET

"You are what you eat." I've heard that saying many times, but it never made much of an impact until I began changing my diet in the process of treating my own chronic sinusitis. I'm now convinced that most chronic medical conditions can be helped significantly by a healthy diet. With specific regard to the sinuses, the change I recommend most is to avoid milk and dairy products. They tend to increase and thicken mucus secretions. If you would like to compensate for the loss of calcium in your own or your child's diet, the following foods are especially rich in calcium: broccoli, kale, sesame seeds and sesame seed butter, tofu, and soy cheese. Or you can buy a liquid calcium and magnesium combination at most health food stores.

Sugar and caffeine should also be avoided because of their depressant effect upon the immune system, and especially if you're suspicious of yeast causing your sinusitis. A nutritionist once asked me, "Would you fill the gas tank of your car with sand?" She felt that filling your body with sugar is equally destructive. Sugar not only has no nutritional value, it's also harmful. Caffeine is a drug to which most Americans are addicted. It is a stimulant that races our engines for a few hours, only to leave us with a greater sense of fatigue when the effect wears off. The quick fix for this state of low energy is simply to drink another cup of coffee or tea or another bottle of soda pop. Your whole body, not just the immune system, suffers as a result of being on a perpetual "roller coaster." The best way to break this addiction is to do it very gradually, substituting noncaffeinated beverages. Please be aware of the possible withdrawal symptoms of headache, fatigue, and irritability.

I'm sure most of you are familiar with the recommendation to decrease your consumption of red meat and egg yolks. These are both substantial sources of cholesterol, which is a major contributor to heart disease. Alcohol should be consumed only in moderate amounts (two to three beers, or one cocktail, or a glass of wine per day). Studies have shown that complete abstainers from alcohol have a slightly shorter life expectancy than those who drink in moderate amounts. However, if a yeast infection is a possible cause of your chronic sinusitis, don't drink any alcohol. Since sugar and alcohol seem to be major dietary contributors to the problem of yeast, it's not difficult to understand how the typical American diet has encouraged this widespread infection.

Try to decrease your consumption of food additives. These include chemical preservatives (e.g., BHA, BHT, sodium nitrite, and sulfites), artificial colors, and artificial sweeteners (e.g., saccharin, aspartame [Nutrasweet], and cyclamates). Almost every one of these additives has been shown to have a potential health risk.

Perhaps our biggest problem with food is our appetite. Americans eat far too much, and obesity has become an epidemic. A massive nine-year U.S. study on caloric intake involving two dozen laboratories, sixty government and university researchers, and 24,000 rats and mice is currently in its fifth year. The results of restricting caloric intake by 40 percent have had a dramatic impact on increasing longevity. The most prominent advocate of human caloric restriction is Roy L. Wolford, M.D., an immunologist at the University of California at Los Angeles, who has raised some of the world's oldest mice using caloric restriction. He has written about his findings in his books *Maximum Lifespan* and *The 120-Year Diet*.

Well, now that I've eliminated many of your life's greatest pleasures—ice cream, soda pop, sugar, coffee, and alcohol—as well as 40 percent of your calories, I hope you're still with me. Our society has chosen food as its greatest treat, and unfortunately, the foods that are the most highly prized not only have no nutritional value but can ultimately make us sick. I'm sorry. I can tell you that when I stopped eating ice cream nearly five years ago, I thought it would be a lot more difficult than it turned out to be. What happens is that shortly after making these dietary changes, you will begin to appreciate new rewards—more energy, less mucus, fewer pounds, and a great feeling of accomplishment that comes from applying self-discipline toward doing something beneficial for yourself. Remember, too, that these are just recommendations, not commandments. My own guideline on this subject (and on many others, for that matter) is "Everything in moderation, including moderation." I do believe, however, that if you're miserable with sick sinuses you should try to adhere as closely as possible to these suggestions.

I realize that I've kept you in suspense long enough before telling you what is acceptable to eat. What's left? A healthy diet is one that is rich in fruits, fresh vegetables, whole grains (e.g., brown rice, bulghur wheat or kashi, oats, millet, quinoa, lupina, whole wheat noodles), and fiber (e.g., bran cereals, beans, apricots, and prunes). Good sources of protein are nuts, seeds, fish, turkey, chicken, and the soybean products tofu, tempeh, and saitan. The foods that are most strengthening to the immune system are also most beneficial to the sinus sufferer with nasal allergies. They are garlic, onions, and citrus fruits.

This is only a brief discussion about nutrition. Attending classes on the subject or consulting with a nutritionist would allow you to tailor a healthy diet to your personal tastes. Through my own investigation, I've concluded that a macrobiotic diet appears to provide the best nutrition with the lowest liability. Macrobiotic means "large (view of) life." It implies taking responsibility for your health by living and eating according to your daily physical condition, level of activity, and climate. It is based to some extent upon Hippocrates' axiom "Food is medicine, and medicine is food." Some good books on this subject are *Natural Foods Cookbook* by Mary Estella and *Introduction to Macrobiotic Cooking* by Wendy and Edward Esko. The book that seems to be the most recommended by nutritionists is *Food Is Your Best Medicine,* by Henry G. Bieler, M.D.

In Chapter 2 I mentioned the foods that most commonly produce the allergic reactions that can cause chronic sinusitis. If you have followed the above recommendations without a noticeable improvement in your condition, then I would try eliminating all of these foods from your diet for at least three weeks: cow's milk and all dairy products, wheat, chocolate, corn, white sugar, soy, yeast (brewer's and baker's), oranges, tomatoes, bell peppers, white potatoes, eggs, garlic, peanuts, black pepper, red meat, coffee, black tea, beer, wine, and champagne. I realize how difficult this can be, but it need only be for three weeks. Then begin to reintroduce each of these foods into your diet at the rate of one every three days. It should then be obvious to you which food, if any, your body is sensitive to. If you're suspicious of food sensitivities, or suffer from hypoglycemia or chronic fatigue, then *High Energy,* by Rob Krakovitz, M.D., is an excellent resource.

I wish there were some way to make dietary change both

simple and easy. If there were, I'm sure it wouldn't have taken so many years for my family's diet to have reached the point it has, and that's with my daughter Carin eager to be a vegetarian. If there is a good health food store not too far from your home, try to shop there. The salespeople can begin to educate you. They're usually very helpful. Many supermarkets now have health food sections. Take a few extra minutes on your next trip to see what looks good. Be a little adventuresome, but do try to implement change very gradually. This should not be done in two weeks. Those who take their time have a much greater chance of maintaining their healthy diet. Although there are many powerful therapeutic measures that I will describe in this part of the book to help your sinuses, none may be more valuable than eating only food that is nourishing to your body.

WATER

Water has been called our most essential nutrient. Regular water-drinking may be the simplest, least expensive self-help measure for the maintenance of good health.

The percentage of water in a human body varies from 60 to 80 percent. A baby at birth is about 80 percent water, and the average adult is between 60 and 70 percent water. Every function of our body occurs in a water medium. Water helps to cleanse the blood by removing wastes through the kidneys; it is vital to digestion and metabolism; it carries nutrients and oxygen to the cells through the blood; it helps to regulate our body temperature through perspiration; it lubricates our joints; and as I have already mentioned, it is needed for the respiratory tract to work most efficiently as it lubricates the mucous membrane. The sinuses can more easily drain when you are well hydrated.

Yet many Americans are chronically dehydrated. This can impair every aspect of the body's normal functioning. It can result in excess body fat, poor muscle tone and size, decreased digestive efficiency (constipation), increased toxicity in the body, joint and muscle soreness (especially after exercise), and water retention (the body retains water to compensate for the shortage). This is why proper water intake is important for weight loss.

A healthy but nonactive adult weighing 160 pounds should drink about ten eight-ounce glasses of water per day, or one-half ounce per pound of body weight; an active, athletic person of the same weight should drink thirteen to fourteen eight-ounce glasses per day, or two-thirds ounce per pound. Try to spread your intake throughout the day (it's best to drink between meals), and don't drink more than four glasses in any given hour. Don't substitute beer, coffee, tea, soft drinks, or fruit juice for pure water. Although they all contain water, they also have other ingredients that can negate the positive effect of water. Herbal tea, natural fruit juices (without sugar; they should be diluted 50 percent with water), and some soups (low salt, no sugar, the clearer and thinner the better) can become a portion of your daily water requirement. Often overlooked is the fact that we also obtain water by absorbing it through our skin while bathing and showering.

Water quality is so variable in the United States that it is impossible to generalize about whether you should drink tap, bottled, or filtered water (I don't recommend distilled water for drinking). Some communities don't even have to treat their water, while others have high levels of lead and radon, the two worst contaminants. Radon can cause cancer, and lead can impair the development of brain cells in children. According to Gene Rosov, president of WaterTest Corporation, the nation's largest independent drinking-water testing laboratory, "the majority of the health-related risks that are present in drinking water are a result of the contamination added *after* the water leaves the treatment and distribution plant." This means that it would be a good idea to have the water at your tap tested, regardless of what your local water utility claims about water quality. You can call your health department for a referral for testing.

It is a fact of life in America today that we can never know for certain whether what we drink or eat is completely safe. Do the best you can—remember to drink more water, make it convenient (keep a water container in your car and at your desk while working), don't wait until you're thirsty, and most importantly, be sure that there's always a bathroom nearby.

VITAMINS, HERBS, AND
NUTRITIONAL SUPPLEMENTS

In case you hadn't noticed, living in urban America can be extremely stressful. Almost daily we are exposed to chemical stress, emotional stress, and infection. Each type of stress has numerous sources. For instance, chemical stress can come from polluted air, polluted water, pesticides, insecticides, heavy metals, and worst of all, radioactive wastes. The primary way stress harms us is by weakening our immune systems with highly toxic molecules called free radicals. According to Deepak Chopra, M.D., the author of *Quantum Healing: Exploring the Frontiers of Mind/Body Medicine*, free radicals are the "metabolic end-products in the body of environmental pollution, food toxins, carcinogens, and emotional toxins." Denham Harman, M.D., of the University of Nebraska says, "Today it seems very likely that the assumption that there is a basic cause of aging is correct and that the sum of deleterious free radical reactions going on continuously throughout the cells and tissues is the aging process or a major contribution to it."

Medical research has already implicated free radicals as causative factors in many diseases, e.g., arthritis, mental disorders, and heart disease, as well as in susceptibility to infection and in the process of aging. In fact, over the past thirty years, research has revealed a common factor in every single degenerative disease of our time—cell damage due to free radicals.

The most common free radicals are produced as by-products of oxygen metabolism, and they are responsible for most of the cellular damage. Fortunately, our bodies manufacture antioxidant enzymes within the cells for protection against free radicals, and also employ antioxidant nutrients (e.g., vitamin A [beta-carotene], vitamin E, and vitamin C) supplied by our diet. As long as there is an adequate supply of oxygen, water, antioxidant nutrients, and enzymes in the body, cell damage is minimized. When any one of these is deficient, cell damage is accelerated, as in the process of aging and/or disease. Through their critical role in helping to prevent disease, vitamins, acting as antioxidants, can offer considerable help to our body's immune system.

In chronic sinusitis and other diseases, the cells are being overrun with an excess of free radicals and our immune system cannot maintain its protective shield. This occurs when the stresses in our lives lower our·body's production of anti–free radical substances (antioxidant enzymes) to a level less than our needs. Unfortunately, living in cities makes it difficult to avoid most of our stressors. It is a wonder that the majority of us are still "healthy," i.e., free of a chronic disease. For those who have not been as fortunate, and for anyone else interested in strengthening their body's natural defenses, practicing preventive medicine, or experiencing a greater degree of physical health, the following recommendations for vitamins, herbs, and nutritional supplements will help.

VITAMIN C

In 1970 Linus Pauling, a Nobel Prize winner, began publishing his findings on the benefits of megadoses of vitamin C in the prevention and treatment of colds. The verification of his findings by other researchers has been complicated primarily by the great variability in the dosages and types of vitamin C that have been used. In my experience, vitamin C has been extremely effective in the treatment and prevention of both colds and sinus infections. Since colds are the most common cause of acute sinusitis, if you can prevent them you will be practicing very good preventive medicine for sinusitis.

The average daily dose for prevention is 3000 milligrams (mg), and if you have a cold or sinus infection (acute or chronic) I would recommend as much as 15,000 mg per day. This amount should be taken in divided dosages, either 5000 mg three times per day with meals (to avoid stomach upset, it is best to take most vitamins with food) or 2000 to 3000 mg every two to three hours. As another option, you can also take time-released vitamin C that lasts for twelve hours. Most other vitamin C tablets last for only six to eight hours. This high dosage for colds and sinus infections should be maintained for about one week or until your symptoms begin to improve. Then begin to taper the dosage very gradually over the next two weeks to get back down to the usual daily dose of 3000 mg. Possible side effects of high-dosage (above 3000 mg) vitamin C are diarrhea, bowel gas, and cramps. If you experience these symptoms, cut back on your next dose by 1000 mg. Another less common side effect is the development of kidney stones. This can usually be prevented by drinking the recommended daily amount of water or by taking 75 mg of vitamin B6 per day.

Another method for taking vitamin C is called "titrating to bowel tolerance." It was developed by Robert Cathcart, M.D., who has treated over 9000 patients with large doses (some as great as 100,000 mg per day) of vitamin C. The maximum relief of symptoms is obtained at a point just short of the amount which produces diarrhea. According to Dr. Cathcart, the amount of vitamin C which can be taken orally without causing diarrhea when a person is ill sometimes is over ten times the amount he or she would tolerate if well. Using this method he has successfully treated a host of viral infections (e.g. colds, influenza, mononucleosis, and viral pneumonia), environmental and food allergies, cancer, rheumatoid arthritis, hepatitis, and yeast infections.

There is quite a variation in the strength of different brands of vitamin C. For instance, 1000 mg of one brand may be much better absorbed than 1000 mg of another. Such differences usually result from combining the vitamin C with minerals such as sodium, calcium, zinc, or magnesium. The salesperson at your health food store should be able to help you choose the best one. There are two vitamin companies that I am aware of that make high-potency vitamin C, Nutri West and Natrol, but they are not the only ones. Taking vitamin C in a powder will also help increase absorption.

Vitamin C, as an antioxidant, is a free-radical scavenger. Our bodies can use a lot more of it when we are under stress. Use your own discretion in varying your daily dosage depending on the degree of stress you think you've experienced that day. If it was a high air pollution day or you had a rough time at work, take more than the 3000 mg. The same recommendation holds true for all the other vitamins and herbs I will mention in the following sections. Vitamin C and all the others are more effective if eaten in the foods that have high concentrations of them rather than taken in pill form. The foods highest in vitamin C are red chili peppers, red sweet peppers, green sweet peppers, kale, parsley, collard greens, turnip greens, mustard greens, broccoli, brussels sprouts, cauliflower, guavas, oranges, canteloupe, and strawberries. These foods are better (for vitamin C content) when eaten raw rather than cooked.

Vitamin C appears to be the vitamin most important for good health. In addition to being an antioxidant, it is essential in the manufacture of collagen (a tough, fibrous substance necessary for wound healing); it also has an antiinflammatory capacity, especially in some autoimmune diseases such as lupus and rheumatoid arthritis; it facilitates the absorption of dietary iron; it enhances the immune response and white blood cell activity; in conjunction with vitamin E, it strengthens arterial wall "cement" and provides greater protection against cholesterol buildup and heart disease; and in at least one study it was used successfully in the treatment of AIDS.

VITAMIN A AND BETA-CAROTENE

The major sources of vitamin A are found in the form of its precursor, beta-carotene, which is converted to vitamin A in your gastrointestinal tract. Beta-carotene is a member of the family of carotenoids, substances usually found in foods that are yellow, orange, or red. It is found primarily in the following foods (listed in roughly descending order of vitamin A content): carrots, sweet potatoes/yams, kale, spinach, mangos, winter squash, cantaloupe, apricots, broccoli, romaine lettuce, asparagus, tomatoes, nectarines, peaches, and papayas. Vitamin A itself can be obtained directly from cod liver oil, liver, kidney, eggs, and dairy products.

Vitamin A helps to maintain the integrity of mucous membranes, is required for growth and repair of cells, is necessary for protein metabolism, protects night vision, and protects against cancer. Beta-carotene has been shown to have an effect as an anticancer nutrient—a discovery made by the Japanese more than twenty years ago. It is also a powerful antioxidant and a potent immunostimulator. In recent research conducted by Charles Hennekens, M.D., of Harvard Medical School, beta-carotene was found to dramatically reduce (by 50 percent) strokes and heart attacks in people who already have cardiovascular disease. Adequate beta-carotene in the diet should supply the vitamin A you need, but vitamin A deficiency in the United States is not uncommon. According to a survey by the U.S. Department of Health, Education, and Welfare, about 60 percent of women and 50 percent of men have intakes below the standard set for good nutrition. Vitamin A can be toxic to the liver in prolonged dosages greater than 50,000 I.U. (international units) per day, but beta-carotene is not. The only side effect of high doses of beta-carotene is yellowing skin, which is not dangerous and disappears when levels are reduced. For sinus infections it is recommended that you take beta-carotene 50,000 I.U. two times per day. After the infection (acute or chronic) has been resolved, this dosage can be cut in half and continued indefinitely.

VITAMIN E

The specific functions of vitamin E are unclear. It has recently been recognized as an antioxidant and in some studies has been shown to raise levels of HDL cholesterol (the desirable kind). For people with sinusitis, 400 I.U. of vitamin E daily are recommended. This dosage need not be reduced as the symptoms of the infection subside. Foods highest in vitamin E are crude and unrefined soybean oil and wheat germ oil, fresh wheat germ, whole grains, raw nuts (most varieties), and all green leafy vegetables.

MULTIVITAMINS

There are so many comparable multivitamins from which to choose that I would allow the salesperson at the health food store to direct you. Make sure your choice has all of the B vitamins. Take one daily whether you have sinusitis or not, and in addition to the vitamin supplements A, C, and E.

MINERALS

The two minerals that seem to be most effective in aiding the body's immune system are selenium and zinc. In a recent article in the *Journal of the National Cancer Institute*, men with lower levels of selenium in their blood were most likely to develop cancers of the lung, stomach, and pancreas. Low selenium levels may also be linked to bladder cancer, in addition to contributing to causes of asthma. For sinus infections (to be taken only when you have symptoms) I recommend either selenium citrate, aspartate, or picolinate in a dosage of 195 micrograms (mcg) daily; or take selenium in a combination pill with vitamin E. Foods high in selenium are whole wheat products, fish, whole grains, mushrooms, beans, garlic, and liver. Selenium can be toxic to the body, so don't maintain a dosage greater than 100 mcg for longer than two weeks.

Zinc appears to be critical to the release of vitamin A from the liver and is vital to the whole process by which new cells are produced and protein metabolized for repair of body tissues. People with sinusitis should take zinc picolinate or oratate 15 mg three times per day, only when symptomatic. The foods highest in zinc are beef liver and turkey (dark meat).

HERBS, BOTANICALS, AND OTHER REMEDIES

It has been estimated that nearly 25 percent of all pharmaceutical drugs are made from plants, herbs, leaves, bark, or roots. In September 1990, cancer researchers asked the Department of the Interior for federal protection for the Pacific yew, a tree found in the ancient forests of the Pacific Northwest whose bark provides a scarce new cancer-fighting drug. The fact that we are destroying global forests so rapidly, especially the rain forests, means that we are eliminating potentially life-saving drugs without even knowing it. Many species of plants are becoming extinct before they have been studied by botanists to determine their value. There are still a few human cultures remaining that depend almost entirely on naturally occurring vegetation for their medicines.

Onions, the herbs garlic, echinacea, and goldenseal, and bee propolis all seem to strengthen the immune system to such an extent that they might be called natural antibiotics. I recommend all of them to patients with both acute and chronic sinusitis (types 1 and 2). They can be taken in addition to a pharmaceutical antibiotic in the form of a capsule, liquid, or tea. Good reference books for medicinal herbs are *A Textbook of Natural Medicine*, by Joseph Pizzorno, N.D., and *The Complete Botanical Prescriber*, by John Sherman, N.D.

Garlic is a member of the lily family. It is a perennial plant that is cultivated around the world and has been used throughout history to treat a variety of ailments. Egyptians have been using it for almost 5000 years and the Chinese for at least 3000 years. Hippocrates and Aristotle cited many therapeutic uses for garlic including the relief of coughs, toothache, earache, dandruff, hypertension, atherosclerosis, hysteria, diarrhea and dysentery, and vaginitis. It is effective as an antibacterial, antiviral, antifungal, antihypertensive, antitumor (especially uterine tumors), and antiinflammatory agent. It is for the most part nontoxic, with the exception of causing bad breath. Many brands of garlic are available at health food stores in pill, capsule, and liquid forms. The ones that claim to be odorless have unfortunately removed the key ingredient in the garlic that fights infection. I no longer recommend those.

Echinacea is at the top of the list of immunity-enhancing herbs. A perennial herb native to the American Midwest, its properties include immunostimulator, wound healer and antiinflammatory, antiviral, antibacterial, and antineoplastic (cancer). It can be taken alone or in a liquid combination with goldenseal, in a dosage of forty drops three times per day. It also comes in capsules. Think of echinacea as you would an antibiotic. It must be taken regularly in order to have a therapeutic effect.

Goldenseal is a perennial herb native to eastern North America and is cultivated in Oregon and Washington. It is best known for its action in soothing inflammatory conditions of the respiratory, digestive, and genitourinary tracts caused by allergy or infection. It acts as a tonic for the mucous membranes. Goldenseal should not be taken by women who are pregnant or who plan a pregnancy in the near future. There is also considered to be a minimal risk to children and people over fifty-five with the use of goldenseal, and it should not be taken in large quantities for extended periods of time. With acute sinusitis, you can take twenty to thirty drops three times per day.

Bee propolis is an extract from the bee's body (it is *not* bee pollen), and it comes in both liquid and capsules. The dosage is 500 mg three times per day. If you use the liquid form, follow the instructions on the bottle. Bee propolis appears to strongly enhance immune function.

There are a growing number of products available containing the herb ephedra, a natural decongestant, from which many of the pharmaceutical decongestants have been derived. The following products (with the name of the company in parentheses) contain ephedra in combination with other beneficial herbs: Sinustop (Nature's Way), HAS (Nature's Way), and Sinus-Ade (Dr. Clayton). There are others. One that does not contain ephedra but has many other medicinal herbs helpful for both sinusitis and allergies is Cobiozin (Great Life Lab). After selecting one of these, you should follow the dosage instructions on the package.

Recently several vitamin companies have introduced products that combine many of the antioxidants with other medicinal herbs. If any are available at your health food store you may be able to fulfill the above recommendations with just one kind of tablet or capsule.

For readers whose primary complaint is a terrible postnasal drip, or just lots of clear nasal mucus drainage without a sinus infection, I've recently learned of an effective remedy. It's fish oil. It can be found in the store as Super EPA (300 mg). Begin with a dosage of two or three capsules per day, then add one per day until your symptoms have improved. If you are deficient in fish oil, and therefore a good candidate for this treatment, you might have several of the following symptoms: dry eyes; dry mouth or thirsty a lot; easily cold; easily overheated; dry skin everywhere except face and scalp, which are too oily; cracking on sides of heels and fingertips; breaking of fingernails (in layers); rough skin on thighs, buttocks, and backs of arms. The most common side effect of this treatment is belching fish oil. This can be minimized by refrigerating the capsules and taking them cold. Diarrhea and a flu-like syndrome are also possibilities. Fish oil has also been found to be effective for the treatment of arthritis and chrònic urticaria (hives).

For those people whose sinuses suffer primarily as a result of nasal allergies, I would recommend all of the above vitamins, with lesser amounts of the minerals and herbs, and in addition, a natural antihistamine called Antronex. It can be taken twice per day, and if your health food store doesn't have it, they may be able to order it from the manufacturer, Standard Process. You might also add vitamin B6 200 mg twice per day and pantothenic acid 500 mg three times per day following meals.

Two other natural remedies for chronic sinusitis are peppermint oil and camphorated salve (Tiger Balm). I put a very small amount (one drop is enough) of peppermint oil on my fingertip, then wipe it around the *outside* of both nostrils. The oil, which acts as a stimulant, seems to improve circulation to the nasal and sinus mucous membranes. This enhances the effect of breathing clean and moist air. I like to spray my nose with the saline spray or stand in front of the humidifier and then apply the peppermint oil. It feels wonderful! Eucalyptus oil has a similar effect. The Tiger Balm seems to work on the same principle for your lungs. With a sinus infection I recommend applying it to your chest two or three times per day.

EXERCISE

No discussion of physical health would be complete without including the subject of exercise. Americans live in a relatively sedentary society. We watch an average of more than four hours of television every day; only 36 percent of our children are required to take physical education classes in school. The majority of adults give lack of time as the most common reason for not exercising. Studies have shown that sedentary people, on average, don't live as long or enjoy as good health as those who get regular aerobic exercise—brisk walking, running, swimming, cycling, or similar workouts. Some researchers now believe that getting no exercise may be a more significant risk factor for decreased life expectancy than the combined risk of cigarette smoking, high cholesterol, overweight, and high blood pressure.

The word "aerobic" literally means "with oxygen," and it refers to prolonged exercise that requires extra oxygen to supply energy to the muscles through the metabolizing of carbohydrates and fat. This is the type of exercise that produces the greatest benefits to the cardiovascular system. The long-term results include slower heart rate, greater cardiac (heart) efficiency, lower blood pressure, and higher levels of physical fitness. If you are looking to quickly improve chronic sinusitis (or any other chronic condition) as well as your overall feeling of well-being, I recommend beginning a regular program of aerobic exercise.

This does *not* have to entail a great deal of time. Keep in mind the factors of fun ("What activity would I like to do?" or "What might feel good to me?") and convenience ("How can this be done in the least amount of time?" or "How can I best fit this into my schedule?"). A minimum program of aerobic exercise need only consist of three thirty-minute workouts weekly, maintaining your fitness heart rate two-thirds of that time. To determine this heart rate, use the following formula: 220 minus your age multiplied by 65 to 85 percent equals your fitness heart rate. For example, a 40-year-old's fitness heart rate is between 117 and 153 beats per minute. You have to know how to take your pulse (using your index and middle fingers, feel the pulse either on the thumb side of your wrist or in your neck just below the jaw) and have a second hand on your watch. Count the number of beats in six seconds and multiply that number by ten to determine your heart rate in beats per minute. When you've attained your fitness heart rate (after about five to ten minutes of exercising), try to maintain it for at least twenty minutes. It is also beneficial to cool down (slower heart rate and less intensity of exercise) for five to ten minutes following the twenty minutes at the fitness rate.

The most convenient forms of aerobic exercise involving the least amount of wear and tear on the body are brisk walking, hiking, swimming, and cycling. If you have easy access to regular cross-country skiing (which most of us do not), you can add that to the list. I no longer recommend running, after seeing numerous patients with running-related complaints, usually involving the knees and feet. In order to cycle year-round, I'd suggest either a good ten-speed with a turbo trainer for indoor cycling or a stationary bike. Treadmill, rowing, stair-climb, and cross-country ski machines also offer an opportunity for excellent indoor aerobic exercise, as do low-impact aerobics classes. There are several sports played one-on-one or in teams, e.g., racquetball, handball, badminton, tennis (singles), basketball, and some others, that have the potential for providing a good aerobic workout. If you live or work where it might be convenient and safe to do (specifically with regard to automobile traffic and outdoor air quality and temperature), then I'd strongly urge you to exercise outdoors. The combination of fresh air and sunshine feels much better than indoor exercise. However, for chronic sinus sufferers and for those trying to practice prevention, air quality is a critical factor in determining where and when to exercise. Ozone is the most harmful of all the air pollutants. It is created by the combination of nitrogen oxides, hydrocarbons, and sunlight. A bright sunny day in the downtown area of most large cities would produce high concentrations of ozone. The EPA considers the air unhealthy when ozone levels top 0.125 parts per million. However, in a study conducted by New York University's Morton Lippman, M.D., thirty healthy adults showed decreases in lung capacity during a half-hour of exercise at ozone levels well below the federal limit.

Writing in the May/June 1989 issue of the journal *Hippocrates,* Benedict Carey suggests scheduling exercise around the rise and fall of pollution levels. In the summer, Carey notes, ozone builds up during the morning, reaches its maximum late in the afternoon, and then ebbs in the evening. In the winter, ozone isn't such a problem, but cold night air can trap a layer of carbon monoxide, nitrogen dioxide, sulfur dioxide, and particulates that may linger into the early morning. A good general practice is to do outdoor exercise in the morning during the summer and in the evening during the winter.

If you're used to walking, biking, or jogging alongside main roads, lung specialists recommend that you stay away from these high-traffic areas during rush hour. Avoid waiting beside stop signs or stoplights, where carbon monoxide builds up.

Henry Gong, M.D., a UCLA pulmonologist, says, "I've seen guys jogging in place next to cars at stoplights. You might as well smoke a cigarette." On windy days pollution disperses quickly as you move away from the road. On calm days it can extend about sixty feet from either side of the road.

If all of these concerns pose too great an obstacle, you live in a highly polluted city, or you're experiencing a wheeze, cough, or tightness in your chest during your workout, then it's time to head indoors for aerobic exercise. Ozone levels in most homes, gyms, and pools are about half what they are outside—even less with a good air conditioning system.

Moderate exercise is less strenuous than aerobic but still beneficial. In a recent research project at the University of Minnesota School of Public Health, moderate exercise was defined as rapid walking, bowling, gardening, yard work, home repairs, dancing, and home exercise, conducted for about an hour daily. A treadmill test determined that those who got this much leisure-time exercise had healthier hearts than those who got less or none. There was no added benefit in doing more than an hour's worth of physical activity. Robert E. Thayer, Ph.D., a professor of psychology at California State University, Long Beach, has found that brisk walks only ten minutes long can increase people's feelings of energy (sometimes for several hours), reduce tension, and make personal problems appear less serious.

For strengthening and toning the upper body, I recommend both push-ups and sit-ups. Remember that with sit-ups you need not raise your trunk any higher than 45 degrees off the floor.

Maintaining and increasing flexibility is an essential part of your overall physical fitness program. Flexibility is the ability to use muscles and joints through their full range of movement. Research has suggested that good muscle elasticity lends agility, a potential for greater speed, and a reduced chance of injury to muscles, tendons, and ligaments. A regular routine of gentle stretching or yoga can be a relaxing and invigorating way to start your day. The books *Stretching*, by Bob Anderson, and *Yoga: A 28 Day Exercise Plan*, by Richard Hittleman, are both excellent guides.

Aerobic exercise was an integral component of the program that I used to cure my own chronic sinusitis, and it is still part of my routine. Initially it requires discipline. Start gradually and try not to push yourself too hard. Exercise does not have to hurt to be beneficial, in spite of the prevailing belief, "No pain, no gain." It won't take long before you'll be looking forward to it as one of the highlights of your day. The benefits that you'll soon realize will help to increase your motivation to continue. You may eventually make it a daily routine, although research has shown no increased cardiovascular benefits beyond five days per week (three times per week is minimum). But exercise does much more than merely benefit your heart. As these aerobic workouts strengthen your heart and lungs directly, your ability to provide oxygen to every part of your body is enhanced—and this, after all, is the scientific basis of physical health. As a human being, you can experience many of life's greatest pleasures only through your body. Regular exercise can add immeasurably to your enjoyment of life and heighten your sense of well-being.

SUMMARY OF
PHYSICAL HEALTH RECOMMENDATIONS

— Follow the treatment program recommended by your physician. This might include antibiotics, decongestants, moisture and irrigation, and any of the other elements of the treatment for acute sinusitis mentioned in Chapter 4.

— Make an attempt to breathe air that is clean, moist, warm, and oxygen and negative ion rich.

— Maintain a diet that is rich in fresh vegetables, fruit, whole grains, and fiber. Avoid dairy products, sugar, caffeine, and red meat.

— Drink about eight to ten eight-ounce glasses of clean water daily, or one-half ounce per pound of body weight, on days you're not exercising. Drink fourteen to sixteen eight-ounce glasses, or two-thirds ounce per pound of body weight, if you're exercising.

— Vitamin C, 5000 mg 3x/day for about one week or until there is a noticeable improvement in your sinus infection, then gradually taper over next two weeks to 1000 mg 3x/day as a daily maintenance dose.

— Beta-carotene, 50,000 I.U. 2x/day until infection clears, then 25,000 I.U. 2x/day.

— Vitamin E, 400 I.U. daily.

— Multivitamin, one daily.

— Garlic,* 2 capsules 3x/day.

— Echinacea + goldenseal,* 40 drops 3x/day.

— Selenium citrate or selenium aspartate,* 195 mcg daily.

— Zinc picolinate,* 15 mg 3x/day.

— Bee propolis,* 500 mg 3x/day.

— Peppermint oil and Tiger Balm, apply 2x/day.

— Aerobic exercise, 30 minutes (at least 20 minutes at fitness heart rate) 3–5x/week. Fitness heart rate = (220 – your age) × 65 to 85%. Exercise can be brisk walking, swimming, cycling, or indoor machines: treadmill, rowing, stair-climb, or cross-country ski.

With the exception of the prescription drugs and most of the herbs and minerals, this is a program that can be continued indefinitely, long after your sinus condition has gone. The vitamins that I still take on a daily basis are 3000 mg of vitamin C, beta-carotene 50,000 I.U., vitamin E 400 I.U., and a multi-

* To be taken only for sinus infections or other acute conditions.

vitamin. I have learned, just as you will, to become much more sensitive to my body. Whenever I feel weak or am exposed to environmental or stressful conditions that are unhealthy to my sinuses, I take several of the vitamins and herbs (or eat more food with these nutrients in them) and increase my dosage of vitamin C.

This approach combines elements of the ''quick fix'' with preventive medicine. I realize that many of the recommendations entail making changes in your daily habits. However, if you're willing to make the commitment and purchase the machines to create healthy air, modify your diet, drink more water, exercise more often, and take the prescribed list of vitamins and herbs, I guarantee that your chronic sinusitis will be vastly improved. I have seen many patients who were able to stop taking long-term antibiotics, decongestants, antihistamines, cortisone, decongestant and cortisone nasal sprays, and asthma medications after adhering to this regimen for several months. Since many of these people had been on their medications for several years, I considered this a quick fix. The patients considered it something close to a miracle. But there is nothing miraculous about it. Physical health is quite basic. It simply entails providing your body with an optimal supply of clean air; healthy food and water; exercise; and extra vitamins to strengthen the body's immune system when it's weak.

Chapter 11

Mental Health

The breadth of the term "mental health" is so great that it almost defies definition. Mental health involves balancing the full development of your capabilities with peace of mind. This requires recognizing the extent to which your thoughts, beliefs, attitudes, and mental pictures limit or expand your potential to enjoy life; learning to make choices based upon your intuition; attaining some degree of clarity regarding your priorities, values, and goals; working at a job that you enjoy; learning to excel at something; and appreciating humor, forgiveness, gratitude, and hope.

As I've already mentioned, it is not within the scope of this book to explore any of these areas in great depth. I would, however, like you to become more aware of mental health and how it might affect your physical status, and to learn some simple things that you can do to attain a greater degree of mental fitness.

BELIEFS, AFFIRMATIONS, GOALS, AND NLP

Most patients who come to see me have already been to one or usually several physicians. Their doctors have told them, "You're going to have to live with your sinus problem"; "You have six months left to live with that cancer"; "Your back/sinus/knee requires surgery"; "There's nothing more that can be done for _____" (the majority of diseases). These statements are, however, only beliefs. They are beliefs based upon the limitations of modern medical science, a highly scientific and technologically advanced approach to the treatment of disease, and they are delivered to the patient by a highly educated individual in a society that defers to academia. These pronouncements, which are in some cases "death sentences," are quickly accepted by most patients and become a part of their own belief system. The vast majority of patients with terminal diseases who accept whatever their doctors tell them ("compliant" patients) die very close to the predicted time. Most of the "difficult" patients who continually challenge their doctors live longer. Bernie Siegel, M.D., in *Love, Medicine, and Miracles*, describes vividly how the beliefs and attitudes of many of his cancer patients affected the outcome of their disease.

Most of the beliefs held by Americans have been defined by the standards, or norms, of our society. But how well does the "norm" fit you, a unique individual? If all of us attempted to conform, the world would be a boring place, devoid of creativity and innovation. We certainly wouldn't be enjoying the ease of living that technology has provided us were it not for many adventuresome individuals who chose to depart from the conventional belief system.

Unfortunately, in every culture there is great pressure to conform. It isn't easy, to say the least, to hold beliefs that run counter to the prevailing wisdom. (I speak from much experience on this subject.) Society, friends, and family all let us know when we stray, with words and phrases like "you should," "you ought to," or—if your belief has created lots of discomfort—"you're crazy!" Most of the time we respond to this pressure by giving up the "unreasonable" or even "outrageous" belief. Ultimately, all of us would prefer to be accepted and loved by others, and "it wasn't that big a deal anyway."

Your belief system has a profound impact on your life—what you eat and think, how you dress and behave, what you do for a living, how you spend your leisure time, what your values and goals are, and how you define health and quality of life. It also determines the nature of the silent messages you give yourself every day. All of us talk to ourselves, and this internal dialogue has a great deal to do with our state of mental health. These messages may be generally self-critical: "You stupid..."; "Why did you say that?"; "Why did you do that?"; "How could you..."; "You should've/could've..."; or they may be more accepting and supportive: "Good job!"; "That's fine"; "You did the best you could." Almost all of my patients are pretty hard on themselves. They are self-critical and pressure themselves to a great extent (time pressure is probably the most common).

As human beings we are imperfect, and all of us make mistakes. It is the way we respond to these failings that creates more or less stress in our lives. Our pattern of response is one we have probably been repeating since childhood. One method of changing the pattern is through the use of affirmations. These are positive statements you can repeat to yourself as often as possible during the day. They should be in the present tense, contain no negative words, and be a response to an often-heard negative message or express a goal you're striving for. For example, if some of the above critical messages sound familiar to you, two affirmations that would help are: "I love and approve of myself" and "I am always doing the best I can." When people begin repeating affirmations, they usually don't believe what they're saying (that's why they're saying them), although they'd like to. In a way, using affirmations is like reprogramming a computer, with your subconscious mind as the computer. The "computer" has been listening to the same message for years, and now you are going to change the input.

The best time to say affirmations is immediately following the negative message. I remember feeling so frustrated with sinus headaches or congestion that I would think or say to myself, "This will never go away." When I began using affirmations, I would immediately follow my hopeless comments with "My sinuses are now completely healed." It always made me feel a little better and gave me some hope, and as my condition improved I began to believe it more and more until it was actually true. Louise Hay has written a wonderful book on self-healing entitled *You Can Heal Your Life*, in which she focuses on the healing potential of affirmations as a means of learning to love yourself. Ms. Hay has recently opened a clinic in Santa Monica, California, for the treatment of AIDS. Her book contains a list of medical conditions, each with a corresponding affirmation. The one for sinusitis is, "I declare peace and harmony indwell me and surround me at all times; all is well." I used that one, too, to help cure my sinus disease.

You can use affirmations to help in changing any belief that doesn't feel good to you, or to help you achieve any goal. Most of the patients that I see have come in because of one or more chronic physical or mental problems. Their objectives are quite clear—"to stop having sinus infections," "to get rid of these allergies," "to have more energy," "to have less anxiety," and so forth. After they have begun to see some improvement in their physical condition, I ask them to make a list of their goals in the other realms of holistic health. I ask them to ask themselves, "What does the ideal future hold for you? What would it look like if you could have all of your desires met?" The answers, e.g., more money, a job that I love, to live in a beautiful place, to be loved, to be understood and appreciated, to have a closer relationship with my spouse, to have a greater sense of the spiritual in my daily life, provide a blueprint for our work together. The answers also give direction to their own self-healing process and become their personal vision. The next step is to write down the answers in the form of affirmations, e.g., "I am living in a beautiful place"; "My job is fulfilling and fun." You must be able to clarify your desires to have any chance of obtaining them. The next step is to believe, however minimally, that it is possible for you to meet these goals. The more you repeat the affirmations the stronger your belief will become.

The third step in this formula for self-realization, an important aspect of mental health, is expectation. The stronger your belief and the more goals you've already manifested in your life, the greater will be your level of expectation. After my chronic sinusitis was resolved, I developed the belief that anything is possible, which has helped me in realizing some of my other dreams. Whatever it is that you *desire*, as long as you *believe* that it's possible, just *expect* it to happen. It is not necessary to know how, or to have a definite plan. Just be patient and flexible and be willing to accept the result even if it arrives in a somewhat different "package" from what you had envisioned. If your objectives are clear, your intuition will help you make the right decisions along the way in getting what you want.

I would schedule a time once or twice a day to recite your list of affirmations. Within a couple of weeks you'll have them memorized and will be able to call upon them anytime a negative belief or message comes up. You may also want to write one or two of them down repeatedly on a daily basis for three weeks. It may sound too simple, but it's actually quite a powerful technique. Remember that you always have a choice as to what you believe.

How you choose to see your sinus condition or any other chronic illness can play a vital role in the way the disease affects you and whether or not it goes away. Some of the more common initial reactions to a chronic or life-threatening disease are denial ("There must be some mistake"); anger and frustration ("Why me?"; "What terrible luck"); self-pity ("I'll never be able to enjoy life again"); and resignation ("I'll just have to put up with it and continue to live this way for the rest of my life"). All of these are quite normal and understandable reactions to something as devastating as a chronic illness. However, if you are interested in healing yourself, it is important to get beyond this point and choose to see your disease in a different light. According to Bernie Siegel, who contributed the following material to the book *Chop Wood, Carry Water* (Rick Fields et al., editors), you have several choices:

— Accept your illness. Being resigned to an illness can be destructive and can allow the illness to run your life, but accepting it allows energy to be freed for other things in your life.

— See the illness as a source of growth. If you begin to grow psychologically in response to the loss that the illness has created in your life, then you don't need to have a physical illness anymore.

— View your illness as a positive redirection in your life. This means that you don't have to judge anything that happens to you. If you get fired from a job, for example, assume that you are being redirected toward something that you're supposed to be doing. Your whole life changes when you say that something is just a redirection. You are then at peace. Everything is okay and you go on your way, knowing that the new direction is the one that is intrinsically right for you. After a while you begin to *feel* that this is true.

— Death or recurrence of illness are no longer seen as synonymous with failure after the aforementioned steps are accomplished, but simply as further choices or steps. If staying alive were your sole goal, then you would have to be a failure, because you do have to die someday. But when you begin to accept the inevitability of death and see that you have only a limited time, then you begin to realize that you might as well enjoy the present to the best of your ability.

— Learn self-love and peace of mind, and the body responds. Your body gets "live" or "energy" messages when you say "I love myself." That's not the ego talking, it's self-esteem. It's as if someone else is loving you, saying you are a worthwhile person, believing in you, and telling you that you're here to give something to the world. When you do that, your immune system says, "This person likes living; let's fight for his or her life."

— Don't make physical change your sole goal. Seek peace of mind, acceptance, and forgiveness. Learn to love. In the process, the disease won't be totally overlooked—it will be seen as one of the problems you are having, and perhaps one of your fears. If you learn about hope, love, acceptance, forgiveness, and peace of mind, the disease may go away in the process.

— Achieve immortality through love. The only way you can live forever is to love somebody. Then you can really leave a gift behind. When you live that way, as many people with physical illnesses do, it is even possible to decide when you die. You can say, "Thank you, I've used my body to its limit. I have loved as much as I possibly can, and I'm leaving at two o'clock today." And you go. Then maybe you spend half an hour dying and the rest of your life living. But when these things are not done, you may spend a lot of your life dying, and only a little living.

I realize that most of you do not have a terminal disease, just a case of good old chronic sinusitis. But each of these options for looking at physical illness can work for you too. In a way they can be seen as preventive medicine, since chronic pain and imminent death, in my experience, have provided the greatest motivation for people to change. Why wait until you've reached that point of crisis?

Another method of changing thoughts and beliefs is neurolinguistic programming (NLP). This is a proven set of mental techniques that were designed by studying people who achieved effectively. NLP was developed in the early 1970s by an information scientist, Richard Bandler, and a linguistics professor, John Grinder, at the University of California, Santa Cruz. From their studies of successful people, they created a way to analyze and reproduce human excellence, resulting in a most powerful practical psychology. NLP can be used to treat a variety of chronic ailments by modifying attitudes and beliefs. It is also effective in transforming phobic and other traumatic responses; helping children and adults overcome reading problems; eliminating unwanted behaviors such as smoking, eating disorders, and insomnia; learning to excel in any area—sports, business, or school; and resolving conflicts between people and within yourself.

NLP can be used as a method of therapy, but it has much broader applications. It's basically a process of teaching people how to use their brains. Most therapy is remedial; that is, directed toward the past. NLP goes much further to study excellence and teach the skills that promote positive change that can generate new possibilities and opportunities. You can use it on yourself to learn a new thinking strategy, change your feelings, change habits, and motivate yourself. There are an increasing number of physicians who are using NLP in their practices. If you are interested in trying this approach, it should not be too difficult to find a certified NLP practitioner in most cities.

WORK

Your job is another vital aspect of mental health. Some of the questions to ask yourself are, "Do I enjoy my job?" "Does my work utilize my greatest talents?" "Is my job fulfilling and challenging to me?" I realize that the answer to these questions for the majority of Americans is no. Unfortunately, there is a significant physical price to be paid for not loving your work. In a recent study on the risk factors for heart disease conducted by the Massachusetts Department of Health, the two greatest risks lay in one's self-happiness rating and level of job satisfaction. Low scores on these two were shown to be better indicators of the likelihood for developing heart disease than high cholesterol, high blood pressure, overweight, and a sedentary lifestyle. The findings were further dramatized by the astounding statistic that more people died of heart attacks on Monday mornings around 9 o'clock than at any other time of the week! Presumably, human beings are the only animals on earth that know the difference between Monday and any other day. The statistic is a striking example of the mind/body connection.

Why, then, do so many of us continue to risk our lives and quality of life (consider also the quality of the air in our work environment) working in jobs that we dislike? The beliefs that are most often responsible are "I have no choice; I need the money"; "I'll never be able to make any money doing what I love to do"; or "I have no idea what I'd enjoy doing or what my greatest talents are." Every one of us has been blessed with at least one God-given gift. For most of us there is at least one activity that we enjoy doing or that we do quite well. That's where you begin the investigation of what your gifts are.

Arnold Patent, in his book *You Can Have It All*, describes in a very clear, logical, and rational way basic universal principles that you can easily apply to obtaining your life's goals. He also suggests an exercise for identifying your gifts. It is as follows:

> Make a list of the things you love to do. Limit the list to those activities that create an excitement in you at the mere thought of them. The shorter the list, the easier it is to reach the desired result. Select the item on the list that is most important to you. Do this no matter how much you may resist picking one item. Remember, picking one does not mean you have to give up the others forever. Make a list of the ways you can express the talent you just selected. It is best to do this daily. Keep a separate book for this exercise. Do not judge the ideas that come to mind as you do this exercise. Write down every idea that occurs to you, no matter how silly or meaningless it may seem. The purpose of the exercise is to stimulate your creative mind. After doing the exercise for a period of time, you will have developed a habit pattern that will continually produce creative ways to express what you love to do. The number of ways you can express yourself by doing what you love has no limit.

The fact that scientists believe that human beings utilize only a small fraction (about 5 to 10 percent) of their brain lends credence to the statement that you have limitless capabilities. You need only to acknowledge that you are seeking a greater level of fulfillment, are willing to change, are ready to take a risk (it could well be a greater risk not to), and begin the exploration that will lead you to work that you love doing. What a wonderful treat it is to give to yourself!

MENTAL IMAGERY

This technique of visualization is one that each of us uses every day, but most of the time it's done unconsciously. Our inner dialogue and the messages we continually give ourselves are very often accompanied by inner pictures. In a sense they are "waking dreams." Since the 1970s there has been a growing interest within the medical and other health professions in harnessing these images to be used as a conscious therapeutic modality. From the pioneering work of O. Carl Simonton, M.D., an oncologist working with cancer patients, to today's growing ranks of physicians who have made mental imagery an integral part of their array of treatment alternatives, the results have been truly astounding. Even more exciting is the fact that the technique easily lends itself to self-healing, as long as you're willing to practice.

Martin Rossman, M.D., from the University of California Medical Center in San Francisco, the author of *Healing Yourself: A Step-by-Step Program for Better Health Through Imagery*, believes that imagery can lead to relief in 90 percent of the problems people bring to their primary care physician. From minor ailments such as back pain, neck pain, arthritis, palpitations, dizziness, and fatigue to conditions as serious as cancer and heart disease, patients can use imagery to address the mental and emotional aspects of their illnesses, thereby helping the physical healing.

I first became aware of mental imagery after hearing on a TV talk show about a nine-year-old boy who had healed his inoperable cancerous brain tumor. He had spent about fifteen to twenty minutes daily sitting quietly with his eyes closed, while picturing missiles being fired into his tumor. The demise of his cancer was documented with brain scans. It certainly got my attention. Shortly thereafter, I had what would turn out to be my last sinus infection. I decided to try mental imagery in addition to my usual regimen for the treatment of acute sinusitis. Without having received any formal training in the method, I sat in a straight-backed chair and focused on deep, relaxed breathing (meditation/conscious breathing will be described in the next chapter) for about twenty minutes. The following vision appeared to me. I saw a large sphere completely covered with a slimy, moldy, greenish-gray crud—terrible-looking stuff! At the top of this globe (if you picture the earth, this would be the North Pole) were a group of about ten little workmen, clothed in overalls and caps, each holding in one hand a very high-powered hose and in the other a long-handled push broom. I watched as they began to methodically work their way down the sides of this sphere while hosing and brushing away the green slime. Underneath was revealed the brightest and healthiest-looking orange I'd ever seen. After the orange was completely uncovered, I got up from my chair and simultaneously felt the largest clump of postnasal mucus I'd ever had in the back of my throat. As I marveled at the size of this mass of greenish-yellow infected mucus in the sink, my sinus infection was almost completely resolved. I've never had another one since. Needless to say, I'm very impressed with the technique, although as this book can certainly attest, it is not the only therapy that I've used to cure my sinus disease.

In addition to treating physical ailments, mental imagery can be used to help you feel more relaxed and peaceful, develop your creative talents, create more fulfillment in relationships, reach your career goals (the clarity of your goal, which I referred to earlier, is definitely enhanced by picturing the goal on a regular basis), dissolve negative habit patterns, and increase your prosperity. If you'd like to learn to use this technique most effectively, I'd recommend either Dr. Rossman's book, or *Healing Visualizations: Creating Health Through Imagery*, by Gerald Epstein, M.D., a professor of psychiatry at Mt. Sinai Medical Center in New York, or *Creative Visualization*, by Shakti Gawain, an extraordinary teacher of holistic health.

OPTIMISM AND HUMOR

It may come as a surprise to learn that an optimistic outlook and a good hearty laugh are beneficial not only mentally but physically as well. As part of the research for their book *Healthy Pleasures*, Robert Ornstein, Ph.D., and David Sobel, M.D., found that the healthiest, most robust people are optimistic and happy and seem to feel that things will work out no matter what their difficulties. As Ornstein and Sobel put it,

"The way they live and envision their lives nourishes their life itself. They expect good things of the world. They expect that their world will be orderly; they expect that other people will like and respect them; and most important, they expect pleasure in much of what they do."

Many of these people seem to maintain a vital sense of humor about life, enjoying a good laugh, more often than not at their own expense. Studies have shown that laughter can improve the function of the immune system. Hearty laughter can be considered a gentle exercise of the body, a form of "inner jogging." Ornstein and Sobel describe the physical effects of laughter:

> A robust laugh gives the muscles of your face, shoulders, diaphragm, and abdomen a good workout. With convulsive or side-splitting laughter, even your arm and leg muscles come into play. Your heart rate and blood pressure temporarily rise, breathing becomes faster and deeper, and oxygen surges through your bloodstream. A vigorous laugh can burn up as many calories per hour as brisk walking or cycling.... The afterglow of a hearty laugh is positively relaxing. Blood pressure may temporarily fall, your muscles go limp, and you bask in a mellow euphoria. Some researchers speculate that laughter triggers the release of endorphins, the brain's own opiates; this may account for the pain relief and euphoria that accompany laughter.

It is possible not only to stay in shape (at least in theory) but also to treat disease through laughter. There is a health center in Arlington, Virginia, called the Gesundheit Institute founded and directed by Patch Adams, M.D.; it focuses on the healing potential of humor. Norman Cousins, in his bestseller, *Anatomy of an Illness*, describes his recovery from ankylosing spondylitis (a potentially crippling arthritic condition), in which he spent a great deal of time watching reruns of "Candid Camera" and movies by the Marx Brothers.

There's some evidence that laughter may strengthen the immune system. In one study, research subjects watching a videotape of the comedian Richard Pryor showed temporarily elevated levels of antibodies in their saliva that help combat infections like colds. Interestingly, the subjects who said they used humor frequently to cope with life stress had consistently higher baseline levels of those protective antibodies.

As Ornstein and Sobel express it, "Laughter is an affirmation of our humanness and an effective antidote to adversity. It can free us to detach and consider problems along new, creative lines. Laughter is a celebration of the unconventional, the unusual, the irregular, the indecorous, the illogical, the nonsensical." It is a powerful medicine and its only side effects are pleasurable. The response I've heard more than once to the question posed to octagenarians, "If you had your life to live over again, what would you do differently?" is "I'd take life much less seriously."

If you are interested in learning a more pleasurable approach to the entire spectrum of holistic health, I know of no greater resource than the book *Healthy Pleasures*. It was even a joy to read.

FORGIVENESS

There may not be a concept more important to mental fitness than that of forgiveness. (I've already discussed this subject to some extent as it relates to beliefs and affirmations.) How often have you thought to yourself, "I am my own worst enemy," or "I sure do make things hard on myself"? Or do you find yourself often blaming others for your own problems or stress? The next time you're aware of blaming someone, physically point your index finger at them (or preferably their image) and take a look at where the other three curled fingers of that hand are pointed. Forgiveness begins with accepting some responsibility for the role you play in shaping your life's experiences. You cannot practice forgiveness on anyone else before starting on yourself. The affirmations "I am always doing the best I can" and "I acknowledge and accept that I am the creative power in my world" are both helpful in learning to forgive yourself.

Stephen Levine, in his book *Healing into Life and Death*, devotes an excellent chapter to forgiveness. It begins with the following sentence: "The beginning of the path of healing is the end of life unlived." It also contains a "forgiveness meditation" that I often recommend to my patients.

Albert Ellis, Ph.D., a psychologist and founder of the Institute for Rational-Emotive Therapy in New York City, has probably done more psychotherapy sessions than any other psychologist—some 90,000 hours' worth. The following quote of his, from an article by Claire Warga titled "You Are What You Think" in *Psychology Today* (September 1988), helped me better understand the importance of forgiveness in the spectrum of mental health. Ellis said, "My psychotherapeutic philosophy holds that the vast majority of humans, in every part of the world, are much more disturbed than they have to be because they simply will not accept themselves as fallible, incessantly error-prone humans."

You can learn a great deal about forgiveness by watching or (preferably) playing sports. For example, imagine a tennis player in an important match. Suppose he misses a shot he thinks he should have made. His response can run the gamut from mild disappointment, as evidenced by a facial expression, to obvious rage, with loud self-berating and racquet-throwing. In order to continue to play at an optimal level of performance and remain competitive, he must be able to very quickly forgive himself for having made this bad shot (mistake), since he'll have to make more shots in rapid succession. If he continues to hold onto his anger or his belief that he's a "bad player" for having made a mistake, he will soon lose his confidence, his ability to concentrate, and the match.

This same kind of scenario occurs for most of us on a daily basis, although not usually in the sports arena. Although we may have more time than the tennis player to recover from our mistakes, unless we forgive ourselves and let go of the past, we will lose some degree of confidence, the ability to focus and stay in the present, and the capacity to do as well as we know we are capable of doing.

How, then, does the frequently held belief "I know I did not do as well as I am capable of doing" correlate with the affirmation "I am always doing the best I can"? Given all the circumstances of your life—where and how you were raised; your level of education and training; the present conditions of your personal life and current level of stress—at every moment of every day, you and I and everyone else are always doing the best we can. That is my belief. To me it feels much better than the alternative, and as you practice it on yourself you'll be forgiving others at the same time.

For many high achievers, a capacity for forgiveness has been a critical factor in their success. In order to grow, learn, expand your horizons, and find greater fulfillment in life, you must be willing to change, take risks, and try something new. This cannot be done without making "mistakes," which can also be looked upon as opportunities to learn (just as Bernie Siegel felt illness could be seen as a source of growth). By taking risks you provide yourself an excellent opportunity to practice self-forgiveness. As with anything else, the more you practice, the better you become. "I am always doing the best I can" is not a belief that precludes trying to do better. It allows you the chance to do just that, by helping you to stay in the "game," without destroying your self-confidence. It also makes risk-taking (and life in general) much more fun. If it feels right to you, then why not choose this belief? While you're at it, you can add the corollary, "There are no mistakes, only lessons."

SUMMARY OF
MENTAL HEALTH RECOMMENDATIONS

— Beliefs and affirmations: Identify negative beliefs you'd like to change and put your responses into the form of affirmations. Some that are almost always helpful are:

I am always doing the best I can.

I love and approve of myself.

Everything is happening in perfect time.

I love my body.

For chronic sinusitis, add:

My sinuses are now completely healed.

I declare peace and harmony indwell me and surround me at all times.

— Goals: Make a list of your goals, desires, and objectives in every realm of holistic health (physical, mental, spiritual, etc.), as long as you believe that they are even remotely possible. Put them into the form of affirmations and add them to your others to form a composite list. Repeat these regularly either orally or in writing, or record them on a cassette and play them back daily (not quite as effective as the other methods).

— Choice: Recognize that you are a unique individual and can choose your own beliefs based upon your intuition or whatever it is that feels right for you. Choose to accept your chronic illness as an opportunity for psychological growth, for redirection, and ultimately for greater enjoyment of your life.

— Desire, belief, and expectation: These will work to help you achieve any goal. Optimism (the expectation that things will work out well) is also an ingredient found in most healthy people.

— NLP: Helps to change beliefs and attitudes as well as being a method for excelling in any endeavor, e.g., business, sports, or the creative or performing arts. It should be learned from a certified NLP practitioner. To excel in anything can expand your self-esteem.

— Work: Find a job that you love doing and that utilizes your unique talents. Avoid work environments with especially unhealthy air. Do the Arnold Patent exercise described in the text.

— Humor: Look for more humor and opportunities for laughter in your life. Lighten up, and try to take life less seriously.

— Forgiveness: Remember that you are a human being with imperfections, weaknesses, and flaws, and so is everyone else. Learn to accept your mistakes and avoid blaming others. Affirmations can help with this.

A good friend of mine recites the following poem titled ''Thinking'' every night together with his two young sons, just before going to bed:

If you think you are beaten, you are.
If you think you dare not, you don't.
If you like to win, but you think you can't,
It is almost certain you won't.

If you think you'll lose, you're lost,
For out in the world we find,
Success begins with a fellow's will—
It's all in the state of mind.

If you think you are outclassed, you are,
You've got to think high to rise,
You've got to be sure of yourself before
You can ever win a prize.

Life's battles don't always go
To the stronger or faster man,
But soon or late the man who wins
Is the man WHO THINKS HE CAN!

— Walter D. Wintle
Author

Chapter 12

Emotional Health

The emotionally fit individual is one who is aware of his or her feelings and is able to express them. I have heard contemporary American culture referred to as the "no-feeling" society. The feelings are certainly present, but as a result of our lifestyle we have constructed such formidable protective barriers around ourselves that to a great extent we have become unconscious of our feelings.

There appear to be only two basic human emotions—love and fear. The so-called "negative" emotions, i.e., anger, anxiety, depression, envy, guilt, hatred, hostility, jealousy, loneliness, shame, and worry, are all expressions of fear. The feelings of acceptance, intimacy, joy, and peacefulness are all aspects of love. The greater our degree of fear, the less capable we are of experiencing love.

In our culture it is not socially acceptable to express most of the negative emotions, and men especially are not "supposed to" show signs of weakness or insecurity or to cry ("Big boys don't cry"). In a setting where it's not OK to express these feelings, the majority of us have learned over the course of a lifetime to repress them to the point that we are unaware that we even have them. Society has helped immensely with this process of suppressing painful (negative) feelings by perpetuating the myth of a pain-free existence. The myriad of appliances and machines that have eliminated so much of our physical labor; the common use of alcohol or drugs to kill the pain of an awkward social situation or personal crisis; the numerous ads in the media for analgesics—all relentlessly give us a message that not only is pain a bad thing, but that life can be pain free. If we were to spend less time trying to avoid pain, but rather focused our attention on it, accepted it, and relaxed into it, the pain would diminish or even disappear. If we continue to ignore and repress it, it often manifests itself as physical pain, illness, or dis-ease. In fact, chronic sinusitis is most often associated with a tremendous amount of unexpressed anger.

Clyde Reid, director of The Center for New Beginnings in Denver, in his particularly insightful book *Celebrate the Temporary*, says, "Leaning into life's pain can also be a lifestyle, and is far more satisfying than the avoidance style. It requires small doses of plain courage to look pain in the eye, but it prepares you for more serious pain when it comes. In the meantime, all the energy expended to avoid pain is now available for the business of living."

I'm not advocating that you go seeking painful experiences. I'm also not proposing that you need to have prolonged or persistent pain. I would call that "suffering." With all due respect to the Buddhists (one of their basic tenets holds that life is suffering), to experience health and happiness you are not required to suffer. I heartily believe that life is to be enjoyed, but the notion that it can be lived entirely without pain is an unhealthy belief. Pain and joy are intertwined, and the more you can allow yourself to accept, embrace, and feel pain, the greater will be your rewards—a heightened sense of emotional health with an abundance of love in all of its expressions.

MENTAL/EMOTIONAL OVERLAP

Although mental health focuses primarily on thoughts, beliefs, attitudes, and imagery, and emotional health has to do with feelings, they are for the most part inextricably related. Most of the methods and techniques described in this section are also beneficial for both your mental and emotional health. For that matter, all the aspects of "mind" (mental, emotional, spiritual, and social) that are discussed in this text are interrelated to such an extent that marked improvement in one area will often have positive ramifications for the others as well. I have separated them not only because they are not exactly the same, but also to enable you to better grasp the scope of each aspect of health and to make it easier to work on each one.

To better appreciate the mental/emotional connection, I will return to Albert Ellis (Claire Warga, *Psychology Today*, September 1988) and the following statement: "My basic assumption is that virtually all 'emotionally disturbed' individuals actually think crookedly, magically, dogmatically, and unrealistically.'' David D. Burns, M.D., is the director of the Behavioral Science Research Foundation and acting chairman of psychiatry at Presbyterian Medical Center of Philadelphia. His latest book is *The Feeling Good Handbook: Using the New Mood Therapy in Everyday Life*. He writes,

> Certain kinds of negative thoughts make people unhappy. In fact, I believe that unhealthy, negative emotions—depression, anxiety, excessive anger, inappropriate guilt, etc.—are *always* caused by illogical, distorted thoughts, even if those thoughts may seem absolutely valid at the time. By learning to look at things more realistically, by getting rid of your distorted thinking patterns, you can break out of a bad mood, often in a short period of time, without having to rely on medication or prolonged psychotherapy.

Burns offers the following checklist of thought distortions:

— All-or-nothing thinking. You classify things into absolute, black-and-white categories.
— Overgeneralization. You view a single negative situation as a never-ending pattern of defeat.
— Mental filter. You dwell on negatives and overlook positives.
— Discounting the positive. You insist your accomplishments or positive qualities "don't count."
— Magnification or minimization. You blow things out of proportion or shrink their importance inappropriately.
— Making "should" statements. You criticize yourself and others by using the words "should," "shouldn't," "must," "ought" and "have to."
— Emotional reasoning. You reason from how you feel. If you feel like an idiot you assume you must be one. If you don't feel like doing something, you put it off.
— Jumping to conclusions. You "mind read," assuming people are reacting negatively to you without definite evidence for this. Or you "fortune tell," arbitrarily predicting bad outcomes.
— Labeling. You identify with your shortcomings. Instead of

saying, "I made a mistake," you tell yourself, "I'm such a jerk...a real loser."
— Personalization and blame. You blame yourself for something you weren't entirely responsible for, or you blame others and ignore the impact of your own attitudes or behavior.

It is now widely accepted that negative thoughts and their subsequent feelings contribute to physical illness. Conversely, recent research has revealed, positive emotions actually produce substances in the body that are identical to the ingredients of pharmaceutical drugs used to help people feel better. For example, when you feel peace and tranquility, your body makes molecules identical to those in the tranquilizer Valium. When you feel exhilarated, the body manufactures interleuken-2, a powerful anticancer drug. Considering the fact that each dose of pharmaceutically produced interleuken-2 costs almost $40,000, if you were to engage in an especially fun-filled activity, your body could probably produce millions of dollars' worth of this drug while helping you prevent cancer.

PSYCHOTHERAPY

Traditional psychotherapy, based upon Freudian principles and the practice of psychoanalysis, has been the conventional medical approach to the treatment of mental and emotional disorders. Just as with the rest of traditional medicine, it is a disease-oriented approach, where patients turn to be "fixed." The majority of patients seeing psychiatrists are labeled with a psychiatric diagnosis and treated with psychotherapeutic drugs. The arsenal of these drugs is constantly expanding as medical research continues to explore the physiology of the human brain. In fact, Prozac, one of the newest antidepressants, has quickly risen almost to the top of the list of most prescribed drugs in this country. The trend in psychiatry is very definitely moving in the direction of less counseling and more drug therapy, although every one of these drugs has potentially unpleasant side effects. The emphasis is on treating the symptom with drugs rather than encouraging the patient to learn methods of changing attitudes or behavior, or just be with their pain and learn from it.

A distinct exception is the rapidly expanding field of cognitive therapy. As a therapist and theorist, Albert Ellis has been a a pioneer in this relatively new branch of psychotherapy. It stresses the importance of cognitions—ideas, beliefs, assumptions, interpretations, thinking processes—in the origins and treatment of emotional disturbance. There are many different types of cognitive therapies, all of which teach people how to evaluate critically their own thought processes to solve their emotional problems and to learn to trust in their own reasoning ability, rather than adhering to the standards and norms of others and of society in general. It is based upon the power of people to transform their current beliefs. Unlike the Freudian approach, the focus is not on the past but on the present. *If you can change what you think, you'll change the way you feel.* In a society that looks for fast solutions, this "brief" form (usually less than a year) of psychotherapy takes much less time than the traditional psychotherapeutic approach.

The job of counseling is increasingly being assumed by a group of psychotherapists that includes psychologists, social workers, pastoral counselors, and anyone else with a counseling degree. The health care industry, particularly the medical insurance companies, has helped to create the changes that are occurring in this field. They discourage long-term psychotherapy by only reimbursing for a certain number of visits to the therapist; by paying for only a portion of the fee, with a large copay assumed by the patient; or by not paying for this service at all.

Although this book is intended to be a self-help guide, and holistic medicine focuses on self-healing, I strongly advocate psychotherapy as an important means of improving your present state of holistic health. In addition to the obvious mental and emotional benefits, physical effects have now also been documented. In a study conducted at the UCLA School of Medicine by Norman Cousins involving two groups of cancer patients, the group that had psychotherapy for one and a half hours per week for six weeks showed profound positive changes in their immune systems. The group that received no counseling had no change in their immune function. More and more therapists are becoming aware of the connection between psychotherapy and spiritual growth, and have incorporated spirituality into their therapeutic program. Ideally I would seek someone to work with who has made this transition and understands and appreciates the importance of spirituality in the healing process. I'd also recommend someone who practices cognitive therapy. The therapist should be someone with whom you feel comfortable and can relate to. It would be prudent to interview several before selecting one.

As I've mentioned before, goals are extremely important. Try to clarify what it is you're looking to achieve in psychotherapy, and be as specific as possible. The greater your clarity, the shorter your therapy. However, you might very well be in such emotional pain that drug therapy sounds very good to you, and that may be just what you need. Find a psychiatrist and get started. You also have the option of seeing a holistic physician. It should be apparent from this text that psychotherapy is one aspect of such a physician's job.

There are times when the symptoms of dis-ease can be so overwhelming in one particular aspect of health, whether it's physical, mental, etc., that you can feel almost paralyzed or suicidal. Your life seems to be at a standstill and you feel worthless and/or hopeless. You must determine your own threshhold of discomfort and when it has been reached, seek help in a way that feels best to you. This is your program, and no one knows you better than you do. In order to continue to work on a balanced approach to holistic health you cannot allow yourself to get "stuck" in one area for too long. Try to learn something from each experience, then move on. In some instances that can take a year or more. Whether it's the death of a loved one, a divorce, a business failure, or a chronic or terminal disease, you must go through a period of grieving and adjust to your loss. Elisabeth Kubler-Ross, M.D., has identified five stages in this process—denial, anger, bargaining, depression, and then acceptance. Allow yourself to feel all of your feelings and know that there is something to be gained from this experience. Realize that however miserable you feel, it is only temporary. Remember that to live without pain is not to fully experience life.

MEDITATION AND BREATH THERAPY

If we as a society do not allow ourselves to feel, then what is it that we're doing to avoid our feelings? Workaholism may be the most common means of "escape." Our minds are so busy with "important" thoughts that there is neither room nor time for feelings. Another means of escape, drug abuse, has become such a threat to the stability of our culture that President Bush has declared a "war" on drugs. That's fine, but it is only another example of symptomatic treatment. With all the publicity and billions of dollars being spent on this campaign, I have never heard any government official question why so many millions of people have been willing to risk their lives to avoid confronting their feelings. Our extremely fast-paced society and the "quick-fix" syndrome are other symptoms of avoidance. We are fascinated with fast and easy solutions to satisfy our needs for food, sex, money, energy, entertainment, exercise, transportation, communication, and health.

Why the hurry? Where are we running? To make more money or to stimulate our minds to a greater extent? Our quest for money, power, material wealth, recognition, and intellectual superiority have all become major distractions in our society, and, in many instances, addictions. Life could be so much more profitable and infinitely more enriching if we would just SLOW DOWN! You can "smell the roses" (they're always available) or simply tune in to life—to the messages your body continually gives you, to what you're thinking and feeling, to the value of your relationships, to your connection to the earth and to your fellow human beings.

One way to effectively slow down is to learn to breathe more consciously. This may be the least of breathing's beneficial effects. As I've discussed earlier, oxygen is the nutrient most vital to the optimal functioning of the human body. For most people, breathing is an unconscious process that begins at their traumatic entry into this world. There is usually not much more attention given to breath other than to one's ability to maintain this life-given function. The medical profession has not addressed the issue of how man might improve upon this basically unconscious act if it were done in a more conscious manner.

Meditation is one of several disciplines that can be described as conscious breathing. Meditation has several benefits. It slows you down and allows you to obtain more oxygen. It is relaxing (meditation is an integral part of most stress management programs)—it helps to keep you focused on the present, not allowing you to hang on to past regrets or worries about the future. It can empty your mind of thoughts and, if practiced enough, can help to bring more feelings to the surface, allow creative ideas to flow, and heighten spiritual awareness. It is also quite effective in lowering high blood pressure, slowing heart rate, reducing pain (especially headaches), and as an adjunct in treating heart disease and many other physical ailments.

Ideally meditation should be practiced in a quiet place, sitting on the floor cross-legged or in a chair with feet on the floor and the back unsupported. Abdominal breathing is done through the nose at a rate of approximately three full breaths (inhale and exhale) in one minute. In abdominal breathing, with each inhalation your abdomen protrudes and with each exhalation it flattens. To practice, place a hand on your belly. To stay focused on the breath and not get distracted by your thoughts (they'll be there, but just let them come and go), it can help to repeat (silently) a very short affirmation or just one word (e.g., "love," "peace," or whatever you'd like) on both the inhalation and exhalation. Initially try doing it for five minutes a day, then gradually increase the time to twenty minutes twice a day. Another technique you could try is to count slowly and silently to five ("one thousand one, one thousand two," etc.) on the inhalation, hold your breath for a count of five, exhale for five, then pause for five before beginning the next cycle. Don't be discouraged if this doesn't come easily. Sitting and breathing without thinking, listening to music, or obviously accomplishing something is not the easiest exercise for most Americans to master. I can assure you, though, that if you continue to practice, you will soon begin to appreciate the many benefits of this simple routine. The next time you feel especially stressed, try to pay attention to the way you're breathing. Your breaths will probably be shallow and irregular (people tend to hold their breath when they're anxious). This would be an ideal time to give a five-minute meditation a try. Meditation can also be a good way to start the day (it's energizing in the morning) and as a means of unwinding after work or before bed (it's relaxing later in the day). Many books are available on the subject of meditation. One that I would recommend is *A Gradual Awakening*, by Stephen Levine.

There are quite a few varieties of breath therapy, sometimes referred to as "breath work." What they all have in common is the ability to help you become more aware of deeply held and often painful feelings. Breath therapies are similar to meditation in their focus on the breath with the objective of emptying the mind of thoughts, but they differ in the type of breathing. Most breath therapies use the technique of "connected breathing," which is much more rapid than the breathing of meditation. Each inhalation immediately follows the exhalation of the preceding breath. Mouth breathing is usually recommended, and both abdominal and chest breathing are used. The therapy can be performed even more effectively under water with the use of a snorkel. Two of the more popular breath therapies are rebirthing and holotropic therapy (with loud music accompanying the breathing). I would suggest attempting breath work only under the direction of a skilled breath therapist. Because of the emotional release that results from this work, such individuals often include psychotherapy as a part of the process. The therapist I have worked with is supervised by a psychiatrist. Although the field is still in its infancy, breath therapy is already being recognized by many physicians as a powerful therapeutic modality for emotional health.

DREAMS AND JOURNALING

According to Robert Langs, M.D., a psychoanalyst and chief of the Center for Communicative Research at Beth Israel Hospital in New York City, "Dreams are extraordinarily reliable commentaries on the life you really live—the people you care about, the events you anticipate, the problems you are trying to solve. Every dream reflects an unconscious response to an emotionally charged situation in waking reality. [Dreams] consistently point out aspects of your feelings that you have overlooked, ignored, or tried to keep at bay. My own studies have indicated that the very process of remembering a dream promotes emotional stability. Analyzing dreams is an extremely helpful way of maintaining your equilibrium and your emotional balance" (*New Age Journal*, July/August 1988).

There are at least two primary obstacles that prevent us from easily using our dreams as a tool for better emotional health. Most dreams are quickly forgotten, and the few that we do remember are filled with symbolism and imagery that do not lead to simple interpretation. Dr. Langs believes that it is more natural to forget a dream than to remember it, because of our unconscious efforts to protect ourselves from undue mental and emotional pain. He thinks that we have unconscious intuition and that we should trust it. "When the conscious mind is ready to cope with the meanings embedded in a dream," he comments, "in most instances you will dream some other version of it later—and remember it." I was relieved to learn that, since I've been able to remember very few of my dreams and have felt some frustration at not being able to benefit from the wealth of emotional feedback they contain.

If you are able to recall some of your dreams and would like to use them in your self-healing process, I would suggest keeping a pad and pencil or a tape recorder by your bed. By writing dreams down or verbally recording them immediately after you awake, you'll be able to retain more of the details. The more often you do this, the better you may be able to understand the symbolism of your dreams. There are psychotherapists (usually with a Jungian orientation) who are quite skilled in dream interpretation and can help you. There are also three books that I'd recommend: *Do You Dream?*, by Tony Crisp, which offers many alternative interpretations of symbols; *The Dictionary of Symbols*, by J.E. Cirlot; and *What Your Dreams Teach You,* by Alex Lukeman. A dream, however, is a highly personal experience, and the dreamer is ultimately the only one who can appreciate its deepest meanings.

Journaling is the written recording of your feelings, thoughts, and any other information you'd like to clarify for yourself. If journaling is done on a regular basis it can increase self-knowledge tremendously and be both enlightening and enlivening. In a sense you become your own therapist or your own best friend. Instead of talking or trying to convey what you're feeling to another person, you're writing to yourself. Communicating with yourself this way seems to allow for greater clarity and ease, probably because there is much less concern about judgment—you are the only one who will be reading what you write, and you don't have to worry about spelling or grammar. In the book *Opening Up,* James W. Pennebaker, Ph.D., effectively documents the benefits to one's physical health that can be gained by writing about upsetting or traumatic experiences. If you write on a regular basis, your journal can become an emotional "diary." There is a highly technical method of journaling referred to as "Progoff," which would have to be learned in a class or through reading the book *At a Journal Workshop*, by Ira Progoff. I don't think that's necessary to be able to benefit from this technique.

EMOTIONAL RELEASE

In American society today the two most recognized emotional ailments are anxiety and depression. Although it is not established as a separate diagnosis, I have found anger to be a primary component of both, especially the latter. In fact, many psychiatrists believe that repressed anger is the "fuel" for depression. Although it is not always apparent to individuals suffering from sinus disease, it has become clear to me that anger is almost universally present both as a causative factor and as an element that helps to maintain chronic sinusitis.

Anger is a perfectly normal human emotion. We usually feel some degree of anger on a daily basis. But anger has been stigmatized in this country, and it is not usually acceptable to express it. Much of the negative attitude toward anger has to do with fears about how much the expression of this strong feeling will affect or be perceived by others. We're often afraid that our anger will hurt someone else's feelings, or that we may be perceived as harsh, abrasive, offensive, cruel, or even emotionally unstable. Comments such as "He's in a rage," "She really flew off the handle,'' or ''Don't go near him, he's having a fit'' help to reinforce our fear of expressing anger. Much of the time we repress it so quickly and unconsciously that we may not even be aware that we feel anger. I have seen many people who have ''practiced'' this conditioned response for most of their lives, beginning with early childhood, and are so adept that they have no awareness of what they've been doing.

The medical profession has endorsed psychotherapy as the best means for adolescents and adults to deal with ''excessive'' anger and fear (i.e., depression and anxiety, along with a host of other emotional disorders). The psychotherapeutic vehicles for treating these conditions are drug therapy and counseling. Both are mental or mind-focused tools. The drugs directly affect the brain, and counseling to a great extent is a verbal and intellectual exercise that can take years to complete.

In recent years many psychotherapists have begun teaching their clients a multitude of methods using sound and their bodies to quickly and effectively release anger. Not surprisingly, the most common of these techniques is screaming. It certainly worked well when we were young kids. The most difficult problem involved with screaming is finding a place where you won't attract attention or be considered crazy. Doing it in the basement of your home, in a closet, or in the car with the windows rolled up are all possibilities. If you want to make less noise you can hold your hands over your mouth when you scream. Take a deep abdominal breath just before screaming, and try to have the sound come from your diaphragm or deep in your chest, not from your throat (in order to protect your vocal cords). Slowly move your upper body or trunk from side to side and up and down while you're screaming (this will be a real challenge if you're sitting in your car). Two or three screams in succession are enough.

Punching is another effective method for venting your anger. I bought a heavy punching bag and boxing gloves and make daily visits to the basement for just a couple of minutes of punching. I do it preventively on a regular basis rather than waiting until I'm in a rage. However, when I do feel a lot of anger, punching is a great way to release it. Instead of a punching bag, you can also punch pillows or your sofa with your fists or with a baseball bat or broomstick.

For those of you with young children, the Yogi Bear Bop Bag might be a good way for them to learn the same thing. You could not only accept and approve of their anger, but encourage them to pretend that the Bop Bag is either you or their brother or sister or whomever it is they are angry at. A family physician friend of mine has done this with his children and it works quite well. What a gift of emotional health to give your kids—to let them know that it's OK to be angry and provide them with an acceptable means of expressing it.

Another technique involves stamping the floor with your right foot (first raise your knee waist high) while simultaneously bringing your right arm across your chest, elbow bent, and then forcefully bringing it back to its original position just as your foot hits the floor. This movement is accompanied by a grunt (an accentuated exhalation). Then repeat the same thing on the left side. Continue alternating sides for three to four minutes. When you've finished you'll feel a bit tired but much more relaxed. All of these anger-releasing techniques—screaming, punching, and stamping—should be done as you exhale.

I had one patient who interrupted me as I began explaining anger release to her and told me, "I don't have a problem with that. I go to K mart and buy some of their least expensive glasses, and whenever I get really angry I throw some of them against a brick wall and I feel much better."

If none of these physical methods interests you, then try talking to yourself or expressing your anger to your spouse, another family member, or close friend, as long as the anger is not directed at them. Whatever feels comfortable to you is fine, but choose something and try it. Anger release has been extremely helpful for sinus sufferers.

Screaming is not the only method of emotional release that we left behind in early childhood. For men especially, crying is a luxury not often indulged in (in our society men cry only one-fifth as often as women). There are "oceans" of tears that Americans have not allowed themselves to shed. Yet recent evidence from tear researcher William Frey suggests that the tears produced by emotional crying (as opposed to those triggered by injury or physical pain) may help the body release stress and dispose of toxic substances. They also contain endorphins, ACTH (adrenal hormone), prolactin (ovarian hormone), and growth hormone, all of which are released by stress.

The vast majority of people report that crying improves mood and offers a welcome release of tensions. At least one study of men and women with peptic ulcers or colitis showed that they were less likely to cry compared to their healthy peers. These patients were more likely to regard crying as a sign of weakness or loss of control. It may not be easy at first, but if you feel the tears coming, try to let go and allow them to flow. It's a very healthy thing to do, both physically and emotionally.

PLAY

Along with screaming and crying, play is another thing that many of us have relegated to childhood. As a means of expressing joy, passion, exhilaration, and at times even ecstasy, play is an essential component of emotional health. The notion that play is something to be abandoned as soon as you "grow up and get a job" is an unhealthy belief. In fact, if you've found a job that you love doing, then work and play can become almost indistinguishable. As George Halas, former owner of the Chicago Bears football team, once said, "It's only work if there's someplace else you'd rather be."

Whether or not you've been able to experience work as play, I'd strongly advocate that you find at least one activity other than work that you thoroughly enjoy. In America, we live in a recreational paradise. Even so, there are still many adults who have never given themselves the opportunity to play. Our public schools do a barely adequate job of teaching this "secondary" skill. Some private schools, which require all students to participate in sports and strongly encourage involvement in theater, art, and music, are much better in this respect. Boy and Girl Scouts are good, although play isn't their primary focus, and most summer camps are even better.

I recommend either sports, games, and other activities requiring some body movement, or active creative pursuits such as dance, playing a musical instrument, acting, singing, painting, crafts, or gardening. Although I realize that many people derive great pleasure from playing cards or chess and other board games and from collecting (e.g., stamps, coins), these are primarily mental exercises. In our society, we already spend most of our time exercising our minds. To create a healthier balance, we should be looking for activities that utilize our bodies, allow us to better express our feelings, and perhaps even bring us to a greater level of spiritual attunement. Ideally the activity should be something so consuming and absorbing that it requires your total attention. In that way it can provide a pleasurable escape from your normal tension and stress and habitual thoughts.

If you did very little playing as a child, or never developed a hobby or strong interest in any particular recreational activity, choose something that instinctively appeals to you. Then find a good teacher or a class and learn the basics. Be prepared to make mistakes and "look silly." That's part of the risk of doing something new. After that initial first step (the most difficult one), it will be a matter of making a commitment and practicing. The better you become, the more you'll enjoy and appreciate the many benefits of the activity. If you are not interested in learning something new, I'd suggest a simple activity like walking or hiking. What's important is to choose something and try to do it on a regular basis, for at least one hour three times per week.

The importance of play cannot be overemphasized. We live in a culture where work has become our greatest addiction; where achievement, accomplishment, and net financial worth appear to determine self-worth for many. In such an environment, to attain a sense of wholeness and balance it is essential that we regularly let go (at least for a short time) of that responsible, mature, working adult and get back in touch with our playful "inner child."

SUMMARY OF
EMOTIONAL HEALTH RECOMMENDATIONS

— Love and fear: These are the two basic human emotions.

All other feelings are aspects of these. The more of one you feel, the less you'll feel of the other.

— Mental/emotional overlap: Unhealthy, negative emotions, such as depression and anxiety, are frequently caused by illogical, distorted, and unrealistic thoughts.

— Psychotherapy: Choose a psychotherapist carefully from among a group of mental health professionals that include psychiatrists, psychologists, holistic physicians, social workers, pastoral counselors, and anyone else with a degree in counseling. Be clear on your objectives before beginning.

— Meditation: This involves conscious breathing, with benefits in every realm of holistic health. Start with five minutes twice a day and gradually increase to twenty minutes.

— Breath therapy: Any one of a number of methods based upon connected breathing may be used. They're helpful in uncovering deeply held emotions. The method should be learned from a breath therapist.

—Dream interpretation: The very process of remembering a dream promotes emotional stability. Try to record dreams in writing or with a tape recorder as soon as you awaken.

— Journaling: Keeping a daily written record of your thoughts and feelings helps you to become your own therapist and best friend.

— Emotional release: Practice at least one anger release technique daily. Most are physical methods that include screaming, punching, hitting, and stamping. Crying can improve your mood, release tension, and remove toxins from the body.

— Play: Select a sport, game, activity, or creative pursuit requiring body movement. Try to practice it for one hour three times per week. Allow yourself to become more childlike.

Chapter 13

Spiritual Health

Before beginning, I would like to make it quite clear that this is not a discourse on religion, although it is based on truths common to all religions. Spiritual health means to me a heightened awareness of a power greater than oneself. This higher power can be referred to as God, the Creator, the Source, Infinite Intelligence, Jesus, Adonoi, Yahweh, Allah; or your inner healer, voice, teacher, guide, child, or higher self. Whatever term feels most comfortable to you is the right one. Through balancing the metaphysical with the material, a program of spiritual fitness will allow you to more consciously access this higher power. The result will be a profound reduction in your degree of fear and an increased capacity to love unconditionally both yourself and others. Additional benefits might include reversing heart disease (spiritual health is an integral part of Dean Ornish's treatment program) and eliminating substance abuse (spirituality is the basis of the Twelve-Step programs used for alcohol, drug, and other addictions); it's also great for healing sick sinuses!

Each of the world's great religions prescribes a method for gaining greater awareness of God (I'll use this term since it's the one most commonly used). Each believes that theirs is the one correct path to spiritual enlightenment. Yet three of them believe that there is only one God (so although there are different names, it must be the same one), and there is a single moral principle expressed as the essence of all of these faiths.

Buddhism: Hurt not others in ways that you yourself would find hurtful.

—Udanavarga 5:18

Christianity: All things whatsoever you would that men

should do to you, do ye even so to them.
—Matthew 7:12

Confucianism: Do not unto others what you would not have them do unto you.
—Analects 15:23

Hinduism: Do naught unto others which would cause you pain if done to you.
—Mahabharata 5:1517

Islam: No one of you is a believer until he desires for his brother that which he desires for himself.
—Sunan

Judaism: Thou shalt love thy neighbor as thyself.
—Leviticus 19:18

What is hateful to you, do not to your fellowman.
—Talmud, Chabbat 31a

Along with loving your neighbor, an equally important objective in most of these religions is to love God or to know God. The essence of the Judaeo-Christian doctrine is expressed in the words that Jewish people are instructed to repeat twice daily, "You shall love the Lord your God, with all your heart, with all your soul, and with all your might."

For several thousand years, religions have tried to explicitly tell us what we're supposed to be doing, i.e., do unto others as you would have them do unto you, and love God. What hasn't been quite so clear to most of us is *how* one loves God. Native peoples all over the world, as well as most of our ancestors who lived during biblical times, found their answer by living in harmony with nature. They were agricultural peoples who experienced closeness and felt nurtured by God through their respect and love for the earth.

James Lovelock, Ph.D., in his book, *The Ages of Gaia: A Biography of Our Living Earth*, describes our planet and everything on it as a single living organism. He believes that the dynamic forces that have been shaping the globe for the past 4.5 billion years are continually modifying the environment to allow the survival of all forms of life, guided by an intrinsic homeostatic mechanism. This guiding intelligence was and still is recognized by people living close to the earth as God. Its essence could be found not only in the earth, but in themselves and every other living organism on the planet. This life force is referred to as *chai* in Hebrew and *qi* (pronounced *chee*) in Chinese. This force or life energy is the core of the spiritual component of every human being and is our common bond with our Creator, the earth, our fellow human beings, and all other life forms.

For most people in today's highly technological urban society, science has become God. They have lost any sense of proximity or harmony with the earth, and technology in fact is contributing to its destruction. They expect science to be able to provide them with an abundance of food and water, stimulate their minds, entertain them, allow them to exercise conveniently, solve most of our urban problems, fix the environmental crisis it created, and heal our diseased bodies. But science has restricted itself to the physical, material world that can only be experienced through our five senses of seeing, hearing, touching, tasting, and smelling. It is a world of effects. True causes lie beyond it, in the realm of the metaphysical. Metaphysics is defined in Webster's *New World Dictionary* as "the branch of philosophy that deals with first principles and seeks to explain the nature of being or reality and the origin and structure of the world." It refers to ideas and concepts beyond the scope of our five senses.

Science believes that the universe is ordered and that it obeys the law of cause and effect, i.e., for every action there is a reaction. But the scientific method on its own is incapable of generating new ideas. Max Planck, Ph.D., a physicist, wrote in *Where Is Science Going?*: "When the pioneer in science sends forth the groping fingers of his thoughts, he must have a vivid, intuitive imagination, for new ideas are not generated by deduction, but by an artistically creative imagination." The science of psychoneuroimmunology, a product of this type of creative thinking, is building a solid scientific bridge between the world of the physical and the metaphysical. I'm hoping that this book will enable you to walk across that bridge with me.

To repeat, our modern lifestyle has created a distance between ourselves and the earth and the rhythms of nature. Our spiritual essence, the divine spark or life energy that is within each of us, is transcendent and connects us to all of creation. This concept has been repeated throughout history by almost every prophet and spiritual teacher of every religion. Jesus put it most succinctly: "The kingdom of God is within." Following this line of reasoning, I believe that in contemporary society the simplest and most effective way to learn to love God is to learn to love yourself.

The "self" that I am referring to is not exactly the one that you've come to know. Most of us spend the bulk of our lives tied to a set of traits, which we refer to as "me." We declare, "This is who I am." Psychology refers to this sense of self as the ego, and it is our conscious personality. We spend almost all of our waking time in the ego, and it comprises much of the mental and emotional aspects of the self. But there is still far more to a human being than these components. Brugh Joy, M.D., one of the world's foremost pioneers in holistic medicine and the author of *Joy's Way* and *Avalanche—Heretical Reflections on the Dark and the Light*, offers the analogy of the human ego as a subatomic particle on the tip of a hair on the tail of a dog, wagging the dog. A whole person, including the spiritual component, encompasses a great deal more than the human intellect is capable of comprehending. However, if you choose, there are an infinite number of ways to explore these vast realms of your unconscious and discover a much deeper sense of love and appreciation for the unique individual that you really are. This process can result in a greater degree of unconditional love for yourself and others, and in that feeling lies an experience of God or a power greater than yourself. What follows in this chapter are several methods to assist you on this enlivening journey. To help in clarifying my objective for spiritual health, I often repeat to myself this saying of the late Teilhard de Chardin, a former French priest, "Joy is the most infallible sign of the presence of God!"

MEANING, PURPOSE, AND INTUITION

If you've ever asked yourself the questions, "Who am I?" "Where am I going?" "What am I here to do?," then you have already begun the spiritual journey. Most commonly these questions will arise spontaneously as a result of a heightened sense of mortality, as with advancing age or with a chronic or terminal disease. There are a growing number of people seeking to better understand the meaning of their lives who are neither old nor sick. They may have achieved or have nearly attained their life's goals, or realized the "American Dream," a vision that embraces society's values of financial success, power, material wealth, and recognition. Having achieved all "anyone could ever want," many find it a hollow success. They feel an emptiness that begs the questions "Is that all there is to life?" "Now what?" "Isn't there anything more?" Their life's meaning had been defined by society and was external rather than something that came from within themselves.

For me, the answers to most of these questions began to unfold when I became familiar with the work of Elisabeth Kubler-Ross, M.D. This remarkable woman, a psychiatrist, has been investigating the phenomena of death and dying for most of her medical career, perhaps longer than any other member of the scientific community. The author of the classic text *On Death and Dying* and several other books, she has concluded from her many years of research on this subject that "death does not exist"! She believes that what we call death is merely the shedding of a physical shell housing an immortal spirit; that our time spent in these bodies on earth is but a very brief part of the total span of our existence; and that to live well while we're here means to learn to love.

Initially I was stunned by her words. This was medical science's leading authority on the subject most uncomfortable to physicians (who equate death with failure), and she was making what sounded like some very unscientific remarks. I was unable to dismiss them, however, and in the six years since learning of her conclusions, I have confirmed for myself their validity. Accepting a belief in the existence of spirit and recognizing love as a means of accessing it and its enormous healing potential have helped me to transform not only my medical practice but my life as well. This perspective has provided me with a new direction, goals, and values, dramatically reducing my fear of death and enriching my life beyond measure.

Each of us responds differently to various stimuli. A message that might inspire a greater sense of meaning and direction for one may do nothing for another. What's most important is that you begin asking the questions. If you have taken that first step, then as long as you're patient you'll find what you're looking for. The answers may not come like a bolt of lightning, but perhaps more like a light on a dimmer switch, gradually illuminating a dark or unexplored aspect of your mind. Your guide along this new path will be your intuition. I've heard this inner voice described as ''God talking to you.'' Your progress on this journey of change will be determined by the degree to which you trust your intuition.

The quiet, subtle messages from your intuition have a tough time competing for your attention. Most of the inner messages that you hear come from your ego and are loud, often negative, and fear based (see the section in Chapter 11 on beliefs). But if you learn to listen, you'll begin to hear a ''still, small voice'' from the depths of your awareness. You'll have to slow down, eliminate distractions, and do a lot less talking and more listening if you are interested in developing your sense of intuition. Meditation, conscious breathing, and slow, relaxing (not brisk, exercise-oriented) walks are all helpful methods of learning to listen to this inner voice. All of the remaining sections of this chapter will suggest more ways to enhance this ability.

Learning to follow your intuition is a combination of a life-changing adventure and an enlivening exercise that strengthens your life energy. Just as with any other type of exercise, practice is required. The more you are able to follow that ''hunch'' or ''gut instinct'' or ''deep inner voice'' and experience results that feel good to you, the more you will be able to trust it. This is the foundation upon which faith is built—faith in oneself, God, and the universe. It can become the basis for the belief that the world is really a safe and loving place, where it is OK to trust. If you can learn to trust your intuition, this trust can then extend to the way you interact with the world and can dramatically reduce the amount of stress in your life. This doesn't mean that you will ignore known risks to your health, safety, and security, but it will offer a means of minimizing fear.

There will be instances in which you believe you've been following your intuition and a painful experience results. You quit your old job only to find less satisfaction with the new one; or you move to a new home that turns out to create a lot more headaches than the one you left; or, most commonly, you divorce a spouse and marry someone else with whom you have similar conflicts. These are not necessarily mistakes. They can be seen as lessons. When we were students in school and were given a subject to learn, if we failed we were given a chance to repeat the course. Life can present lessons to us in much the same way, often painfully.

If you are questioning the meaning of your life, it can be helpful to look at some of your most painful experiences. Look at the role you played in each of these instances and how you may have contributed to the situation. Are there some common patterns of behavior? For example, I have been treating a patient for chronic back pain, which at times has been incapacitating for her. Before her first attack, her life was a whirlwind of activity—mother, housewife, PTA, sales job, and aerobics instructor. The back pain made it nearly impossible for her to continue with any of her former responsibilities. As soon as it had subsided, however, she resumed her hectic pace, and within a year the problem had returned. This time it was worse, and it put her out of commission for nearly three months. During this period of inactivity, while lying on her back, she began to appreciate her tremendous desire to achieve, as well as a strong need to give to others. Without the achievements or the ability to give, she felt a sense of worthlessness. Like so many Americans, she did not feel deserving of love unless she was accomplishing at a high level, or taking care of others; she gave very little to herself. She had become a "human doing," and quite a good one at that, rather than taking the time to learn and appreciate what it means to be a human being. Her back has been much better for nearly a year, and she has developed a lifestyle that is much more gentle, nurturing, and healthy. She is able to give more to herself, works only part-time, and as a result is able to spend much more quality time with her family. From this experience she has developed a much greater degree of trust for her intuition as it directs her on a path of caring for herself with more compassion. Taking an exceptionally painful situation and treating it with mercy and acceptance rather than anger and fear will help to bring greater meaning to your life and provide you the opportunity to grow spiritually. *Man's Search for Meaning*, by Viktor Frankl, M.D., a survivor of a Nazi concentration camp, is an inspirational book on this subject.

Another method of finding greater meaning could be to conduct your life as if you have one hour left to live. In a very helpful book on spiritual health, *The Road Less Traveled*, M. Scott Peck, M.D., describes the benefits of living with "death on your left shoulder." This approach quickly and dramatically puts life into a different perspective. It allows you to continually reexamine your values and decide what's really important to you.

Whatever route you take, as you look for meaning you will usually discover greater purpose in life. As previously noted in the Work section of Chapter 11, every individual has at least one unique talent or God-given gift. It is in the expression of this gift that you will often find your purpose. To me, one's purpose has to do with sharing his or her gift with the world and leaving it a better place as a result. I know of no more effective way to realize your purpose than working on a personalized program of holistic health. Several of the student/patients that I've worked with have discovered healing gifts, a discovery that has caused them to shift the direction of their professional careers. Some of life's greatest joys can be experienced in practicing your gifts and in doing what you love to do. (Getting paid for it can be an added bonus.)

PRAYER

Prayer is a spiritual exercise and is the standard Western form of meditation. A national Gallup poll in 1988 found that 88 percent of Americans pray, and most of those who do have more of a sense of well-being than those who don't. A majority say that they experience a sense of peace when they pray and feel that they have received answers to prayers, and more than half say they have felt divinely inspired or "led by God" to perform some specific action. Those polled who said they felt an experience of the divine during prayer are the people who have the highest rating in general well-being or satisfaction with their lives. More than 70 percent of Americans believe prayer can lead to healing, whether it's physical, emotional, or spiritual.

In a study conducted by Dr. Randolph Byrd at the San Francisco General Medical Center, Christians were asked to pray for half of a group of 393 hospitalized heart disease patients; no one was assigned to pray for the other half. The patients were unaware of which group they were in. The results showed that a majority of those who were prayed for needed less medical intervention during their hospital stay than those in the control group.

Since 1968, Herbert Benson, M.D., a Harvard cardiologist, has been conducting research that has conclusively demonstrated that prayer has a multitude of health benefits. He began his research in 1968 on the physiology of meditation, using people who practiced transcendental meditation. They meditated with a mantra, a single word with no meaning to its user (e.g., *om*). Dr. Benson found that the repeated mantra replaced the arousing thoughts that otherwise keep us tense during most waking hours. This resulted in a lower metabolic rate, slower heart rate, lower blood pressure, and slower breathing.

Dr. Benson then studied Christians and Jews who prayed rather than meditated. He had Roman Catholic subjects repeat "Hail Mary, full of grace" or "Lord Jesus Christ, have mercy upon me." Jews used "Shalom," the peace greeting, or "Echad," meaning "one." Protestants used the first line of the Lord's Prayer, "Our Father, who art in heaven," or the opening of the Twenty-Third Psalm, "The Lord is my shepherd." The phrases all worked the same way as did the meditation. Dr. Benson has found that all major religious traditions use simple repetitive prayers. Such repetitions, his research suggests, all create what he calls the relaxation response (RR). This response is exactly opposite to the stress reactions widely studied as the flight-or-fight response, a human being's (or any other organism's) defense against dangers.

As he continued his studies, Dr. Benson found that the benefits of faith may interact with the direct physiological benefits of RR and that prayer sets up the interaction. He also found a connection between RR and exercise—when runners meditated or prayed as they ran, their bodies were more efficient. They were able to achieve greater efficiency by trying to match the cadence of their short prayers to the rhythm of their steps.

Since 1988, Dr. Benson and his colleague, Dr. Jared Kass, a psychologist, have been conducting a series of programs at the Mind/Body Medical Institute at Boston's New England Deaconess Hospital. They've invited priests, ministers, and rabbis to investigate the spiritual as well as the health implications of prayer. *They found that people who feel themselves in touch with God are less likely to get sick—and better able to cope when they do.* They also developed a psychological scale for measuring spirituality both before and after prayer. People high in spirituality, which Benson defines as the feeling that "there is more than just you" and as not necessarily religious, turned out to score high in psychological health. They also have fewer stress-related symptoms. Next, he found that people high in spirituality gain the most from meditation training—they show the greatest rise on a life-purpose index as well as the sharpest drop in pain. Just in case the nearly three-quarters of the American population who already believe that prayer can be therapeutic needed additional confirmation, science has now shown that as it strengthens the spirit, prayer heals the body.

For those of you who already pray, I would certainly recommend that you continue. For those who would like to begin, I'd suggest any prayer with which you might be comfortable or can remember from your religious training. The Lord's Prayer is familiar to most Christians, and the majority of Jews know the Shema and Viahavta. Try to establish a regular routine and repeat the prayer morning and night. You may also have a favorite psalm or passage from the Bible or a prayer book that is especially meaningful to you. Add it to your daily regimen. I've found three psalms in particular to be especially healing. They are Psalm 121, which I repeat every morning; 91, late afternoon or after work; and the Twenty-Third Psalm before bed.

In addition to the prayers and psalms associated with religion and the Bible, you might be interested in more personal prayer. To do this, talk to God as if you're speaking to your best friend and be extremely honest, e.g., "I'm having a problem and I really need some help." It's fine to want things (e.g., money, material things, health, etc.) for yourself or loved ones, but first ask yourself what feeling would result from having the things for which you ask. I'd suggest praying for that feeling rather than the specific things.

GRATITUDE

Most religious traditions prescribe specific prayers or "grace" before meals as a means of thanking God for the food and for our physical sustenance. As with other spiritual practices, there is something to be gained from all of them, or they wouldn't have survived for thousands of years. The more you can appreciate the spirit of the practice rather than merely following the "letter of the law," the greater its value will be. Science is just beginning to appreciate the multifaceted benefits of spiritual practices. As you've just learned with prayer, spiritual practices provide a means of emptying the mind of thoughts and induce the relaxation response. The more you practice, the greater your ability to focus and be present, and the greater the effects.

Feeling grateful can elicit similar life-enhancing benefits. The most spiritual rabbi I've ever met suggested to me the following ritual. As soon as you wake up each morning, before getting out of bed, close your eyes and picture yourself in a scene that makes you feel happy to be alive, or grateful that you've been able to have that experience. You never would have had it if you hadn't lived, and you know that something equally wonderful can happen again. What a great method of creating an attitude of looking forward to each day and appreciating being alive.

Most of us tend to take life for granted. Suppose you choose instead to see your life as a gift you've been given and to be thankful for all that it has provided you—both the pleasures and the pain. As I've discussed, adversity can provide you with the opportunity for tremendous growth. You may not be too happy about it at the time it occurs, but in retrospect you can be grateful for the lessons you've learned.

Gratitude can produce powerful feelings of self-acceptance and joy. It is an attitude that anyone can choose to have, just as you can choose to be positive or negative, be forgiving or unforgiving, see the cup as half full or half empty. It has been my experience that when people choose to look at the up side of life, more positive things start to happen. It seems that we attract whatever feeling we're radiating. When you focus on gratitude, wonderful things happen. It is related to a sense of abundance—you focus on what you do have, not on what you don't have. At the same time you become able to let go of negative thoughts and attitudes.

Just as with almost every other recommendation in this chapter, this isn't easy to do. If you're feeling a great deal of fear and anger, it's especially difficult to superimpose gratitude. But if you can release some of those feelings through forgiveness (see that section in Chapter 11) and acceptance and put your heart into practicing gratitude, I know it will work for you.

As long as you are alive there are always blessings to be grateful for. I rarely go through a day without thanking God for something, and every time I do there is an accompanying feeling of joy.

SPIRITUAL PRACTICES

Most major religions have their own variations on the following practices, but none of them needs to be performed in accordance with any particular ritual in order to be enjoyed. Doing them in whatever way is comfortable for you and creating your own ritual will feel good. The practices that I'll mention involve the four basic elements of our world—earth, air, fire, and water—fasting, and the Sabbath.

EARTH

The earth itself and nature can provide us with a feeling of proximity to God as well as healing energy not found in most congested urban environments. I would suggest spending as much time as possible being outdoors in close contact with the earth, in natural settings—parks, woods, beaches, or mountains. A daily walk is great, or playing a sport, riding your bike, swimming (especially in the ocean, a lake, or a river), gardening, or just finding a quiet or scenic spot to appreciate the beauty that surrounds us.

Roger Ulrich, Ph.D., professor of urban and regional planning at Texas A&M, in 1981 performed a study with the help of Swedish scientists. He showed eighteen students slides of trees, plants, water, and city scenes. The students reported the nature scenes—especially those containing water—made them feel more elated and relaxed; in contrast, the urban scenes tended to elicit sadness and fear. Backing up these subjective responses, electroencephalograph (EEG) readings of the students' brain-wave activity showed significantly stronger alpha waves when viewing the nature scenes—scientific evidence of feelings of relaxed wakefulness.

In 1984, Dr. Ulrich found that exposure to nature speeds recovery from the stress of surgery. When he examined the hospital records of forty-six men and women who had undergone gallbladder operations, those with a window view of a small grove of trees spent about a day less in the hospital than patients with a view of a brick wall. They also required less pain medication and were less upset.

AIR

Try to find a place where the air is reasonably healthy and meditate. See the Meditation and Breath Therapy section in Chapter 12 for specifics on meditation.

FIRE

Throughout the Bible, fire or light is the most prevalent

symbol for the divine essence in man. Being in the presence of an open fire is pleasurable. Anyone who has a fireplace at home and uses it (since wood-burning contributes to air pollution and sinus problems, I'd suggest a gas fireplace) or who enjoys sitting by a fire while camping can attest to it. The simplest and healthiest method is to use candles more often.

WATER

I've already emphasized the importance of drinking it. Now I'm suggesting immersing yourself in it. There is nothing quite so relaxing as bathing in warm water. I'd suggest doing it at least once a day, morning or night. Hot tubs and spas are one of technology's greatest inventions, but if you don't have one, your bathtub will suffice. If you've ever soaked in a natural outdoor hot spring, then congratulations—you've experienced what I consider one of life's ultimate pleasures. Many mineral hot springs can also be quite therapeutic for a variety of ailments. In some that are unimproved (without a cement foundation), you can at times feel so close to nature that it is almost as if you are being enveloped in the womb of Mother Earth.

FASTING

This ancient spiritual purification practice of abstaining from food can have a cleansing effect upon the body. According to the Bible, Moses and Jesus were both able to sustain a fast for forty days. Unless you've attained their level of spiritual mastery, please don't attempt a fast of that duration. I am talking more in terms of one day, during which you abstain from both food and water. Doing this can definitely elicit a heightened spiritual feeling, as it shifts your focus away from physical concerns. Select a day when your work or family responsibilities are limited and you won't be required to be too active. Plan for some quiet time alone, and during the final two hours of the fast drink six to eight glasses of water. This helps to cleanse your body of toxins. See how it feels after you have fasted once or twice, and if you think it's been beneficial, then try fasting on a regular basis, perhaps monthly. You'll be surprised at how much easier it is to do with each subsequent fast.

SABBATH

"Remember the Sabbath day to keep it holy." Although more than 3000 years old, the Ten Commandments remain a worthy set of ethics to live by even in our modern world. To the Jewish people, the Sabbath is still the holiest day on the calendar, even though it occurs every week. It is meant to be a day completely devoted to love—love of God, self, family, and friends. I'm not suggesting that you observe any particular day of the week or even a full day if you can't afford the time. However, for your spiritual health, I'd recommend setting aside the same time each week to indulge yourself in this celebration of life. Try to abstain from anything even remotely resembling work.

TOUCH

As I have said before, there are several topics that don't easily fit into one single component of holistic health but that can create healing benefits in several aspects simultaneously. Touch is one such therapeutic modality. I've included it here because it is not only one of our most effective healers, but within the entire animal kingdom and especially our own species, it might well be the most powerful and direct means of conveying love.

According to Saul Schanberg, M.D., Ph.D., a professor of pharmacology and biological psychiatry at Duke University, "Humans need to touch and be touched, just like we need food and water." Through his research on touch, along with the work of other scientists during the past thirty years, the following findings (as cited in *Hands-On Healing,* John Feltman, editor) have been revealed:

> — In a study involving forty premature infants, half of them were gently stroked for forty-five minutes a day; the other twenty were not. Although all were fed the same amount of calories, after ten days, the touched babies weighed in 47 percent heavier than the unstimulated group. The stroked babies were also more active, more alert, and more responsive to social stimulation.
> — When a person's wrist is gently held by someone else, heartbeat slows and blood pressure declines.

— Children and adolescents hospitalized for psychiatric problems show remarkable reductions in anxiety levels and positive changes in attitude when they receive a brief daily back rub.

— The arteries of rabbits fed a high-cholesterol diet and petted regularly had 60 percent less blockage than did the arteries of unpetted but similarly fed rabbits.

— Rats that were handled for fifteen minutes a day during the first three weeks of their lives showed dramatically less cell deterioration and memory loss as they grew old, compared with non-handled rats.

Yet in spite of the many healthy reasons to touch and be touched by other human beings, we Americans indulge in this simple pleasure very little. One study in the 1960s noted the number of touches exchanged by pairs of people sitting in coffee shops around the world. In San Juan, Puerto Rico, people touched 180 times an hour; in Paris, France, 110 times an hour; in Gainesville, Florida, 2 times an hour; and in London, England, the pairs never touched. The implications and possible causes of this phenomenon would entail a lengthy discussion, although I'm sure the puritanical legacy of associating touch with sex still has a profound effect upon American attitudes. I also agree with William E. Whitehead, Ph.D., an associate professor of medical psychology at the Johns Hopkins University School of Medicine, that a significant part of the blame lies with the father of modern-day psychology, Sigmund Freud. "Freud encouraged austerity in dealing with children. And parents, in an effort to be good parents, bought into that behavior," says Dr. Whitehead. People who aren't cuddled a lot as kids, he adds, tend to develop into nontouching adults. The cycle then repeats itself, generation after generation.

As an osteopathic (D.O.) physician, I learned very early in my medical training about the therapeutic value of the "laying on of hands." Although almost all of our courses and textbooks were the same as those used to train our allopathic (M.D.) brethren, we were taught a more holistic approach to health care that included among other things osteopathic manipulative therapy. This involved soft-tissue stretching (somewhat similar to massage) and adjustments or corrections in the position of the spine and other body parts (similar to chiropractic adjustments). It has taken me a while to realize that the patients responded so well to this treatment not only because of the prescribed techniques, but also because of the healing potential of touch itself. I have also learned of a number of other therapeutic modalities in which touch is a primary healing ingredient. They are acupressure, Alexander technique, applied kinesiology, aromatherapy, Aston-patterning, Berry method, chiropractic, craniosacral therapy, Esalen massage, Feldenkrais method, Hellerwork, hydrotherapy, myotherapy, oriental massage, physiatry, physical therapy, polarity therapy, reflexology, Reichian therapy, Rolfing, sports massage, Swedish massage, therapeutic touch, and the Trager approach. I will not discuss the relative merits of these methods other than to say that all of them deserve to be recognized as legitimate disciplines in the full spectrum of the healing arts.

I have always viewed the practice of medicine as the business of caring. As our health care system continues to change radically, the most insidious shift has been the erosion of the doctor-patient relationship. It has become more impersonal and there is less mutual trust. Within the traditional medical community there is a greater fear of closeness and subsequently less touching of patients except that which is strictly necessary in the course of a diagnostic evaluation. Medical patients may need the comfort of human touch more than most people—a reassuring pat on the shoulder, hand-holding, or even a hug. If caregivers are to do their best job, the powerful healing potential of touch must be learned and has to become a larger component of every physician's therapeutic "black bag."

If you are interested in experiencing a "hands-on healing" technique, I'd suggest trying a practitioner of one of the many therapeutic modalities I just listed. See how it feels and give it a fair trial. If it works for you, that's great. If it doesn't, try something else. Two of these modalities, acupressure and reflexology, I've had experience with in treating chronic sinusitis, and they have both been quite effective. I'll describe them in Chapter 15.

Touch is a gift that you can give to yourself every day. It is merely a matter of allowing yourself to receive and to feel deserving, things that many of us don't easily allow. If you are meditating, praying, or lying in the bathtub, try touching your chest over your heart in as gentle and compassionate a way as you know how. A loving touch is healing, no matter who is administering it.

Animals are perfectly fine sources of tactile comfort, says Alan M. Beck, Sc.D., director of the Center for the Interaction of Animals and Society at the University of Pennsylvania. Numerous studies, he adds, "definitely show that petting an animal can lower one's blood pressure." Other doctors suggest that there are health benefits to be had even from cuddling inanimate objects—teddy bears, for instance. If you have neither a pet nor a favorite stuffed animal, then my prescription for maintaining your spiritual health is to get several hugs daily!

There is no question that we have become too distant from one another. There is clearly a movement in this country to compensate for that deficiency and restore our sense of wholeness and balance. The trend toward more touching is a return to the norms and values of preindustrialized society. Primitive cultures are all very touch oriented. I have lived with one such native group in which touch was the primary method of healing. They believed that their healers had a gift bestowed by God, and that the healing energy that flowed through the healer to the patient was God's love. Whatever it was, I can attest to the fact that the healers' touch worked extremely well for a variety of ailments. By our standards these people might be considered primitive or underdeveloped, but they are clearly much healthier than most Americans in body, mind, and spirit.

SUMMARY OF
SPIRITUAL HEALTH RECOMMENDATIONS

— Spirituality is awareness of a power greater than yourself, most commonly referred to as God. This divine power is the essence of all life on earth and is the spark or life energy within every human being.

— Knowing or loving God and loving your neighbor as yourself are the primary moral principles of most religions. As spiritual health objectives in contemporary American society, they can best be reached through first learning to love yourself. As you do, you will experience less fear in your life and a deeper sense of unconditional love for yourself and others. In that feeling lies a greater awareness of God.

— Meaning, purpose, and intuition: Begin asking yourself what your life is about, where you're heading, and what you enjoy doing. This will help clarify your sense of purpose as well as provide the opportunity to give your gifts to others. Your intuition, or inner voice, is your best guide in this process. Take time to listen and be willing to risk in learning to trust it.

— Prayer: Daily prayers, those prescribed from your religious training and/or personalized "talking to God" prayers, are helpful. I also recommend Psalms 121 in the morning, 91 after work, and 23 before bed.

— Gratitude: Begin your day by visualizing a scene that makes you feel glad to be alive. Don't take life for granted; there are numerous blessings for which to be grateful. Focus on what you have, not what you lack.

— Spiritual practices: Utilize the four basic elements of our world by engaging in outdoor activities that enhance closeness to the earth; meditating or using conscious breathing somewhere with clean air; using candles more often; and soaking daily in a warm bath, hot tub, or natural hot spring. Fasting for one day periodically and observing a regular weekly Sabbath (a day to focus on love, for yourself and others) are both effective practices.

— Touch: This is a basic human need that for most of us is filled far too seldom. There are a multitude of therapeutic disciplines in which touch is the primary healing modality. If you are treating a chronic condition that has not responded to your present regimen, consider choosing one of these approaches. Remember too that hugs heal!

Chapter 14

Social Health

Social health has to do with relationships and our degree of connectedness to other human beings. It involves the balance of autonomy with intimacy. I have found it to be the aspect of holistic health in which we Americans are most deficient, and it is clearly the most difficult for us to work on. The reasons for this social malaise will be a topic for much discussion in the coming decade. I have no doubt that its root cause will be found to be the self-involvement of the seventies and the compelling profit motive, greed, and win-at-all-costs attitude of the eighties expressed by the bumper sticker "He who dies with the most toys wins."

How we created this social dis-ease may become the subject of debates, but the magnitude of its impact upon the foundation of social stability—the family—is unmistakable. As a society we are feeling the pain of a pervasive sense of isolation and alienation, a 50 percent divorce rate, dual-career marriages, stepfamilies, and a generation of adolescents more adrift and alone than any that has preceded them. According to "Turning Points," the 1989 report of the Carnegie Council on Adolescent Development, almost half of all adolescents are at significant risk of reaching adulthood unable to meet adequately the requirements of the workplace, the commitments of relationships in families and with friends, and the responsibilities of participation in a democratic society. They are susceptible to "a vortex of new risks...almost unknown to their parents and grandparents."

It is important to recognize that young people today reflect the world we have shaped for them. What seems dysfunctional in teenagers' behavior may actually be functional ways of dealing with the crazy environment they inherited. What they are mirroring most is our lack of connectedness with others. This sense of separateness can create not only social but physical disease. Dean Ornish, M.D., found that the most common attribute of his heart disease patients was their feelings of hostility and of being apart from others, a sense of isolation. In a study conducted by Kenneth Pelletier, Ph.D., on terminal cancer patients with long-term survival, one of the strongest ingredients in their survival was found to be their relatively high degree of social involvement. The effect of social relationships upon the immune system can also be seen in the high incidence of illness and even death after the loss of a loved one or after moving to a new city, state, or country.

SUPPORT GROUPS

Human beings are socially dependent herd animals, and the quality of our lives has a great deal to do with our level of social integration. (A fascinating look at the human animal can be found in Desmond Morris' *The Naked Ape*.) Human babies have the longest infancy in the animal kingdom. A foal can run within hours of its birth; a kitten or puppy can leave its mother within two months. We humans are born helpless and stay dependent for years. We must bond and be continually cared for or we die. Relatively little of our behavior is programmed by reflexes at birth. Therefore most of our learning, beliefs, attitudes, and world view is shaped by our almost umbilical connection to society. Our need to be a part of a social system does not diminish in adulthood; it actually becomes more elaborate. We look to society to provide food, shelter, goods, information, and health care. It is certainly not surprising that we suffer when the link to others is broken. It also makes perfect sense that medical science has now acknowledged that one of the most therapeutic measures for people with any chronic disease is to join a support group. Whether the condition is AIDS, multiple sclerosis, Parkinson's, or diabetes, there are support groups available in most urban communities. Research has already demonstrated the impressive long-term survival of breast cancer patients who have joined support groups, as well as that of people with heart disease. I was recently asked to speak to the SERI Sinus Sufferers Support System (S^5) at the Solar Energy Research Institute in Denver—the first sinus support group I'm aware of.

There is a definite movement in America toward a greater sense of community. Small (usually less than ten people) support groups for those sharing common values and goals, not just to share the experience of an illness, are becoming much more commonplace. Men's groups, women's groups, and couples groups, sometimes affiliated with a church or synagogue, are forming all over the country for the primary purpose of enhancing spiritual growth while becoming more socially connected. They meet regularly, some weekly, others twice a month, and some monthly. It is a positive and healthy sign of a national social recovery.

MARRIAGE

Marriage can be the most difficult as well as the most rewarding of all relationships. It can be seen as a spiritual practice—most religions regard it as a "holy union." If the basic societal and religious moral principle is to "love thy neighbor as thyself," then its practice begins not with the person living next door, but with the "neighbor" with whom we share our bed.

Marriage incorporates all of the ingredients of a program of holistic health, which is synonymous with learning to love. There is probably not a more effective vehicle for curing sinus disease than to work on your marriage or a committed relationship. The key to success is commitment. It is a commitment to each other and to your growth—both that of the individual and that of the relationship. Once that pact is made, you will begin to recognize that the relationship is an entity that is greater than either of the two of you. As Maggie Scarf says in her book *Intimate Partners*, "When space is provided within the system—space for changing, growing, being different over the course of time—marriage can be the most therapeutic of relationships, the fertile terrain which permits both partners to expand, flourish, and attain their full potentials." Change entails letting go of parts of yourself, and as you do, you'll realize that by giving more to the relationship you are ultimately giving to yourself.

Marriage also promotes physical health. People who are

single, divorced, or widowed are twice as likely to die prematurely as those who are married. This is particularly true of men. Unmarried people also wind up in the hospital for mental disorders five to ten times as frequently. So before deciding upon a divorce, you may want to ask yourselves if you've done all you could do to save the relationship.

After more than twenty-two years of marriage, my wife, Harriet, and I have decided to begin sharing what we've learned with other couples through practicing marriage counseling together. The recommendations that follow have resulted from counseling we have received; from Harriet's master's-level education in social work with certification in marriage and family counseling; from two very helpful books, *Getting the Love You Want*, by Harville Hendrix, Ph.D., and *Intimate Partners*, by Maggie Scarf; and from our many years of working to make our relationship a more conscious one. This brief discussion will contain the methods or exercises we have found to be most helpful. However, if you are interested in making more of a commitment to your relationship, I would strongly suggest that you begin with marriage counseling. As with any new course of study, it doesn't hurt to find yourselves a good teacher.

SHARED VISION

A vision is really a way of defining goals and focusing your energy on their attainment. Without a vision, your relationship can become directionless, and your problem-solving behavior will reflect a crisis orientation. You may have already completed your individual list of goals suggested in Chapter 11. This shared list might include statements relating to the way you feel about each other; where you live; how you play together; how you resolve conflicts; what your sex life is like; and anything else that applies to your situation.

The list that each of you writes should be in the form of affirmations, in the present tense, positive, short, descriptive, specific, and beginning with "we." For example, "We trust each other," "We express our anger toward one another," "We are very affectionate and touch each other daily." After sharing your vision with your partner, combine the similar sentences of both lists to capture their essence and create a new composite list. Try to list the goals in the order of highest value (each of you will rank them differently, so do the best you can). You might also note the ones that will be most difficult for you to fulfill. When you have completed this "mutual relationship vision," schedule a time every day to read it to each other, or record it on a cassette and listen to it together. Do this exercise daily for at least sixty days. This is just one of the sixteen exercises described by Dr. Hendrix in his book. There is also an accompanying workbook available from his Institute for Relationship Therapy in New York City.

LISTENING EXERCISE

Most of us are very poor listeners. It amazes me at times how much we can hear without actually listening. Since communication is the foundation of any relationship, and listening is a critical aspect of effective communication, this listening exercise can go a long way toward creating greater intimacy in your marriage.

Schedule an uninterrupted forty-minute block of time twice a week in a comfortable, relaxed, quiet setting. One person speaks for twenty minutes while the other listens without responding. Then the roles are reversed. The object is to be able to talk freely about whatever you're thinking or feeling without any concern about judgment or criticism from your spouse. In most of our conversations, if we express something that is uncomfortable for our partner to hear we know about it right away. With this exercise the listener will still react to certain trigger words or ideas but will not be allowed to respond. The longer the listener holds on to his or her reaction, the less he or she is actually listening. So the more you practice this, the better you become at letting go of your own thoughts and feelings and at focusing on the art of listening. Some people have described it as being almost a meditative exercise, as it requires you to empty your mind of your own thoughts as you listen.

As the speaker, try not to dwell on the relating of current events, but concentrate more on the feelings these situations have elicited in you. If you're the second speaker, avoid a critique of what your partner just spoke about. In one version of the listening exercise, the couple is not allowed to comment upon anything that was said during the exercise for up to three days following it. For one of the two weekly sessions you might want to try doing it that way. It's definitely more of a challenge, but with even greater rewards. By creating a safe environment for expressing our feelings and allowing ourselves to be vulnerable with our spouse, the listening exercise is an extremely valuable tool for building trust in one another, a much greater degree of understanding and acceptance of each other, and at times exhilarating feelings of intimacy. The last couple to whom we recommended this exercise described their initial reactions like this: "It felt wonderful to have his total attention." "I really liked the fact that she was just listening without giving me any advice."

The listening exercise is described in detail in Maggie Scarf's book.

REQUESTS

When you marry, you enter into a relationship in which you have made a commitment to give love to and receive love from your spouse. Since each of us is different, what feels like love to one person may not even be noticed by another. Most of us attempt to love our partners in ways that feel like love to us, but they may not react as we would. A good method of eliminating this problem is to simply tell each other what feels good to us. To ensure that you receive more of what you want, write three requests of your spouse. These should consist of actions or behaviors that you, the requester, perceive as most loving. Like the affirmations, the requests should contain no negative directions and should be as specific as possible. Some examples might be: I would like you to give me two hugs daily; I would like you to spend one afternoon each week with me; I would like you to buy me flowers once a week; I would like you to help me more with the cooking and cleaning. It can be quite a revelation when someone you have lived with for many years, whom you thought you knew well, tells you what they really would like from you. It may also help to explain your feelings of being unappreciated when actions you perceived as loving were not reciprocated. We often expect our spouses to be "mind readers"—"He should have known what I wanted"; "She ought to have been able to tell how I felt." We really can't know exactly unless we are told. So be specific, get what you want, and make requests. It is extremely important to thank your partner for complying with any request. It usually will not be an easy or natural thing for him or her to do (otherwise you wouldn't have had to ask in the first place), so acknowledge the effort and even greater compliance may follow.

HAVING FUN TOGETHER

The pressures and responsibilities of daily life in America can make it difficult to remember to have fun. For many couples, the glue that holds their relationship together is the memory of enjoyment they shared during their courtship and early years of marriage. To rekindle some of that earlier excitement and sweep away the cobwebs of routine and boredom, it is helpful to regularly schedule fun activities together. Plan a day or half-day each week to spend together away from home in an activity one of you has chosen. Alternate the responsibility for the choice of activity weekly. Being out of the house and going by yourselves can help you focus attention on each other. Choosing something neither of you has ever tried before can add a sense of adventure to your play. If you can manage it, I'd recommend two days per month (an overnight) out of town. You might be surprised at how refreshing and invigorating regular short trips can be for your relationship. Especially if a vacation isn't feasible, these two-day excursions might be just what you need.

PARENTING

Don't expect any quick fix or magic cures in this section. A magician I'm not, just another parent trying to do the best I can. I have no simple approaches to what many see as the most challenging fulltime job in existence. But I do suggest that we can choose to look at parenting as one of life's most enriching experiences; as a chance to play and feel more in touch with our own "inner child"; and as an opportunity to let go of ourselves and experience selflessness. In dealing with our teenagers in particular we are provided with a wonderful vehicle for practicing forgiveness, unconditional love, trust, self-acceptance, self-awareness, and most of all, patience.

A useful guideline in the process of learning effective parenting might be to regularly ask yourself, "Will this (action, response, activity, or demand) of mine help my child's self-esteem?" As is also evident in marriage, *to love another is to help that person better love himself or herself.* Obviously, as human beings, we are not always able to meet this ideal. Children are constantly trying to expand their limits and are testing ours at the same time. While they seek greater independence, our job is to balance our own degree of comfort (encompassing our level of fear, faith, trust, and values) with what would be most beneficial to these young explorers for whom we are responsible. It requires a great deal of awareness to appreciate who these unique persons are and how best to provide them the safety and base of security they need in order to develop their independence and discover their hidden talents and gifts. Most of us take great pride in our children's achievements and strengths and disavow any connection to their flaws. Each of us is a composite of our genetic inheritance from both parents, environmental influences, and the intangible factor of our own human spirit. This combination produces a human being altogether different from any other. As parents we must respect and acknowledge this difference, even though at times we feel as if our children are extensions of ourselves. What we have considered to be good or bad for us might be just the opposite for our children.

In the field of family therapy, the family is usually seen from the "systems" approach. This view holds that if a child's (or anyone else's in the family) behavior is dysfunctional, i.e., harmful to himself and/or others, the problem and the solution lie not solely within that individual but in the whole family system. The use of this perspective encourages parents to look at their role and the partial responsibility that they share for the problem. A child's crisis can be a mirror reflecting to a parent an imbalance in his or her own individual "system" as well as in the family system. One of the significant advantages of family therapy is that change often occurs more rapidly than in individual psychotherapy. In much the same way that holistic medicine refrains from merely treating the physical symptom without looking at the whole person, the systems approach recognizes the need for family therapy when one member of the family is suffering. If this is a situation that applies to your family, I would strongly recommend family counseling.

I have mentioned that anger is a primary cause of sinus disease. The focus of that anger is often either yourself, your spouse, or your children. Now that you know several ways to release it (refer to "Emotional Release" in Chapter 12), there is another way to use anger beneficially, particularly with regard to your children. I have consistently found that the aspects of a child's behavior that upset a parent the most are the things the parent likes least about him- or herself. I guess it's just easier to be angry with our kids than with ourselves. These disturbing behavior patterns become most apparent during adolescence, which merely adds to the challenge of parenting teenagers. For instance, suppose you believe your child has innate ability in a certain sport, with a musical instrument, or in a creative art, but the child refuses to pursue it for fear of making mistakes or looking awkward or silly as a beginner, or perhaps for no reason at all. You feel a very strong reaction, become furious, and find yourself starting to insist that the youngster at least try this new endeavor. Whenever you react so strongly, it's time to stop, reflect, and use the situation as a mirror. Perhaps this particular incident is reminiscent of your own fear of trying new things and might be bringing up feelings of frustration and anger with yourself for the many times you failed to realize your own potential. So, out of anger with your child can arise a chance for you to see yourself more clearly and to forgive and accept both yourself and your child. Opportunities for loving can often present themselves in unusual ways.

Good parenting requires both time and consistency. If you've completed a personal vision list and a shared vision with your partner, they might provide a good idea of what values you would most like to instill in your children. These values can serve as a guide for the rules you both implement and consistently adhere to as parents. Setting limits is just another way of loving your child and yourself.

Time seems to be the ingredient most lacking in today's society. In the typical American family both parents are employed outside the home, and the most striking change for this generation of teenagers is their aloneness. Before adolescence, a high percentage of these children have spent time with many different caretakers, often spending more hours with them than with their own parents. For these and many other reasons, this is not an easy period in which to be growing up in the United States. But even in the two-career household, if the commitment is there, time for the family can be found. Family dinners, for instance, when everyone eats together, are becoming a lost tradition. I'd suggest trying to share at least this one meal together as a chance to converse and get to know one another. Make sure the television is off. The average American watches about thirty hours of TV per week, which must mean that it has become both a distraction and a frequent "guest" at a substantial number of dinner tables across the country.

Other ways to spend time together as a family are to worship together each week at church or synagogue and to designate a regularly scheduled time during the weekend for a fun activity. You can rotate the leader, so that each family member has a chance to choose the activity. The value of play cannot be over-emphasized. Having fun together can sometimes accomplish what many sessions of family therapy were unable to do.

What parents really need to be able to do is show that their love is unconditional, that nothing a child does or fails to do will diminish that love, and that children do not have the power to make or break their parents emotionally by their actions or achievements. That's really all there is to it! Isn't that simple?

ALTRUISM

The late Hans Selye, a pioneer in modern stress research, thought that by helping people you inspire their gratitude and affection, and the warmth that results somehow protects you from stress. That warm feeling may well come from endorphins—the brain's natural producers of euphoria. Even watching others help seems to help us. In a striking study at Harvard University, psychologist David McClelland showed students a film of Mother Teresa, the embodiment of altruism, working among Calcutta's sick and poor. Analyses of the students' saliva revealed an increase in immunoglobulin A, an antibody that can help combat respiratory infections. Even men and women who consciously had no sympathy for Mother Teresa responded with enhanced immunity. Epidemiologist James House and his colleagues at the University of Michigan's Survey Research Center studied more than 2700 people in Tecumseh, Michigan, for almost fourteen years to see how social relationships affected mortality rates. Those men who did regular volunteer work had death rates two and one-half times lower that those who didn't.

The well-researched Type A personality—hard driving, hurried, and competitive—has a higher risk of heart disease than others. In a study performed by Duke University internist Redford Williams, M.D., it was found that the more hostile the person, the more blocked his or her coronary arteries were. At the University of Maryland, James Lynch found that people who do not listen well, who jump at the first chance to answer back, tended to have higher blood pressure.

The evidence is mounting that selflessness not only feels good but is healthy as well. When we choose freely to care, we seem to get as much, or more, than we give. (However, as Ornstein and Sobel point out in *Healthy Pleasures,* being in control and having a choice is crucial to the health benefits of giving: Those who must care for sick loved ones for long periods often report more, not less, stress and illness.)

The closer our contact with those we help, the greater the benefits seem to be. By far my greatest rewards as a physician have come from the gratitude and appreciation I've felt from so many of my patients. Most of us need to feel that we matter to someone. But you needn't be in the healing arts to derive that pleasure. There are a growing number of needy people in our society—homeless, hungry, parentless, and illiterate. There are a multitude of ways to help.

The destructive self-centeredness underlying hostility can be treated with a healthy dose of selflessness. But the treatment works best if your generosity comes from the heart and is not calculated to benefit you. In *Healthy Pleasures*, Ornstein and Sobel devote a chapter to "selfless pleasures." They close with the following:

> Healthy altruism comes from the understanding that you and those around you are part of the same human community or social body. When one person suffers or is deprived, all of us are affected. It is for this reason that religions counsel generosity and service to others. The human community is strengthened and the server, too, benefits.
>
> It is important, even vital, to be able to connect with other people and to be part of life in general; our lives, our health, and our destiny are connected with that of others. The great surprise of human evolution may be that the highest form of selfishness is selflessness.

SUMMARY OF
SOCIAL HEALTH RECOMMENDATIONS

— Social health is defined by our degree of connectedness to other human beings. American culture has bred a society suffering from isolation, alienation, aloneness, and hostility.

— Support groups are small groups of people who meet regularly to share views on common ailments, problems, values, or beliefs, or for the purpose of enhancing spiritual growth. Anyone with a chronic disease or who feels a lack of community should consider either joining or forming a group.

— Marriage is a spiritual practice of learning to love your "neighbor" as yourself, balancing autonomy and intimacy. Some helpful exercises include sharing a vision—listing common goals for the relationship; listening—one partner speaks for twenty minutes while spouse listens without any response, then reverse; requests—make three requests of your spouse for actions or things that would make you feel loved; having fun together—regularly scheduling a block of time for enjoying one another's company.

— Parenting is a challenging opportunity to practice unconditional love on our children as well as ourselves. It requires a balance between teaching independence and allowing the exploration of potential gifts and setting comfortable limits. It takes consistency, time, and the recognition of your child's uniqueness. Try to define your values and establish rules in accordance with them; create time for family dinners and family fun. Parenting may be life's most difficult job.

— Altruism—helping others—can be pleasurable as well as providing a boost to the immune system. Healthy selflessness can be an antidote for the hostility underlying self-involvement. Helping others with genuine goodwill brings a powerful feeling of connectedness, a sense of unity, and the recognition that in giving to others you are ultimately giving to yourself.

Chapter 15

Holistic Specialties

What I have presented in Chapters 7 through 14 is an introduction to and overview of holistic medicine. The material was meant to provide you with some idea of the breadth of this field and give you enough information to begin to practice it on yourself. Conveying the full scope of this healing art would require something on the order of an encyclopedic text.

As a general practitioner of holistic medicine, just as I have been a GP of traditional medicine, I am a "jack of all trades," with a working knowledge of each component of holistic health. However, just as there are medical specialties in various limited areas, there are also a multitude of holistic specialties. Most medical specialties focus on one part or system of the body; e.g., ear, nose, and throat specialists work only on the neck and above, including the sinuses. On the other hand, many holistic specialties encompass all parts of the body but may be limited in the degree to which they address the various components of holistic health. Some holistic specialists focus solely on the physical, others on the mental or emotional. There are those who work almost exclusively on spiritual or social health. The common denominator in most of these healing arts and disciplines is that medical science has not recognized their scientific validity, and therefore they have been largely ignored—in many cases even scorned—by the traditional medical community. In honoring the commitment to heal and teach, holistic medicine involves an openness to complementary concepts as well as an understanding that what is not "proven" is not invalid.

The four holistic specialties that I will briefly present in this chapter are all, in practice, more physically oriented (although in theory they can treat body, mind, and spirit). They are naturopathic medicine, Oriental or Chinese medicine, homeopathic medicine, and reflexology. I've chosen them because I have had personal experience with each one and know that all of them have been successful in treating chronic sinusitis.

NATUROPATHIC MEDICINE

Naturopathic physicians (N.D.s) are specialists in natural medicine. They are trained at four-year naturopathic medical colleges and educated in the conventional medical sciences. They treat both acute and chronic disease. Their treatment modalities come from the sciences of clinical nutrition, herbal or botanical medicine, homeopathy, Oriental medicine, physical medicine, exercise therapy, counseling, acupuncture, natural childbirth, and hydrotherapy. Some naturopaths may choose to combine several or all of these therapeutic modalities, while others may specialize in one specific area.

The basic principles of naturopathy are based upon the concept that the body is a self-healing organism. The naturopathic physician enhances the body's own natural immune response through noninvasive measures and health promotion. Rather than treat the symptoms, naturopaths strive to uncover the underlying cause of patients' diseases, looking at physical, mental, and emotional factors. Health is seen not as the absence of symptoms, but as the absence of the causes of the symptoms. Prevention and wellness are vital principles in naturopathy. These physicians are trained to know which patients they can treat safely and which ones they need to refer to other health care practitioners. As teachers, naturopaths seek to facilitate the growth of patients' responsibility for their own health and to spark the enthusiasm and motivation needed to make fundamental lifestyle changes. The origins of naturopathic philosophy extend as far back as Hippocrates, who stated the principles "Do no harm" and "Let your food be your medicine, and your medicine be your food."

As a distinct American health care profession, naturopathic medicine is almost 100 years old. Early in this century there were more than twenty naturopathic medical colleges. Today there are only two—in Portland, Oregon, and Seattle, Washington. In the 1940s and 1950s, with the advent of more technological medicine, the increased popularity of pharmaceutical drugs, and the belief that such drugs could eliminate all disease, naturopathy experienced a decline. During the past two decades, however, as more people have begun to seek out alternatives to conventional medicine, it has seen a resurgence in popularity.

Naturopathy seems to be making its greatest contributions to the healing arts in the fields of immunology, clinical nutrition, and botanical medicine. Much of the vitamin and herbal regimen for the treatment of sinusitis and the strengthening of the immune system that is described in Chapter 9 comes from naturopathic medicine.

CHINESE MEDICINE

Traditional Chinese medicine is the primary health care system currently used by approximately 30 percent of the world's population. It is believed to be one of the oldest medical systems in existence, dating back almost 5000 years. The practice of acupuncture (a method of using fine needles to stimulate invisible lines of energy running beneath the surface of the skin) is the component of Chinese medicine most familiar to Americans, but the system also includes Chinese herbology, moxabustion (the burning of an herb at acupuncture points), massage, diet, exercise, and meditation.

In ancient China, doctors were not paid if patients under their care became sick. The job of the physician was to keep patients healthy. Chinese medicine believes that a certain process happens before the body develops a problem or disease. A Chinese medicine practitioner (O.M.D.—Doctor of Oriental Medicine) looks for this process or pattern of disharmony. Through questioning, observation, and palpation, a practitioner can determine a person's current state of health and the problems that individual will be at highest risk for developing in the future. In this way Chinese medicine is effective in prevention.

Chinese medicine is based on a history, philosophy, and sociology very different from those of the Western world. Over thousands of years it has developed a unique understanding of how the body works. The Chinese see disease as an imbalance of the body's nutritive substances, called *yin,* and the functional activity of the body, called *yang.* This imbalance causes a disruption of the flow of vital energy that circulates through pathways in the body known as meridians. This vital energy, called *qi* or *chi,* keeps the blood circulating, warms the body, and fights disease. The intimate connection between the organ systems of the body and the meridians enables the practice of acupuncture to intercede and rebalance the body's energy through stimulation of specific points along the meridians.

People who have used Chinese medicine for a particular physical symptom frequently experience improvement in seemingly unrelated problems. This occurs because the Chinese approach tends to restore the body to a greater degree of balance, thereby enhancing the body's self-healing capacity. The whole person is treated rather than just the symptom, and the relationship of body, mind, emotions, spirit, and environment are all taken into account.

The World Health Organization has published a list of over fifty diseases successfully treated with acupuncture. Included on the list are sinusitis, asthma, arthritis, common cold, headaches (including migraine), constipation, diarrhea, sciatica, and low back pain. Acupuncture has also been shown to be quite effective in the treatment of allergies, addictions, insomnia, stress, depression, infertility, and menstrual problems.

Chinese herbs are the most common element of Chinese medicine as it is presently being practiced in China. The herbs are becoming more popular in the United States, but it is still much easier to find a licensed acupuncturist (L.Ac.) than an O.M.D. who is knowledgeable about Chinese herbs as well as acupuncture. Pharmaceutical drugs are usually made by synthetically producing the active ingredient of an herb. Medicinal plants differ from the isolated active ingredients synthetically produced in drugs because they contain associate substances that balance the medicinal effects. Uncomfortable side effects generally come about because the associate substances have been removed. Chinese herbs are capable of regenerating, vitalizing, and balancing the vital energy, tissue, and organs of the body without harmful side effects. They can be taken in pill form or powders or as raw herbs that are made into tea.

Chronic sinusitis can be effectively treated with a combination of acupuncture and Chinese herbs. I'd recommend seeing a licensed Chinese medicine practitioner who has had good experience with herbs. Such practitioners are not that easy to find, but their numbers are increasing as more schools of traditional Chinese medicine are becoming established in this country.

Acupressure works according to the same principle as acupuncture, using the same points on the meridians, but instead of needles being inserted, direct finger pressure is applied to stimulate these points. Of the two techniques, acupuncture is generally more effective, but acupressure allows you to do it yourself. I have included two diagrams here to illustrate the acupressure points you can use for sinusitis (see Figure F).

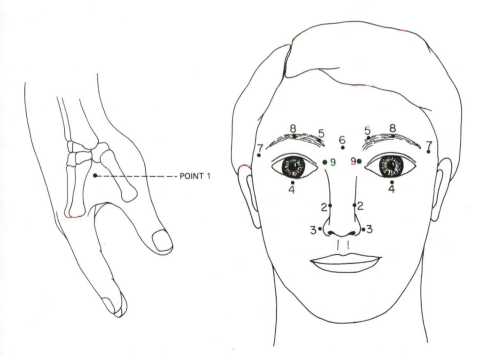

Figure F. Acupressure Points.

Pressure should be applied with your index fingers, with enough strength for you to experience mild discomfort, for about twenty to thirty seconds. This can be done without any finger motion, or you can rotate your fingers counterclockwise. Points 1, 2, and 3 are helpful for anyone with a sinus condition. Points 4 through 8 need only be used if those places are sore to the touch (using mild pressure). Stimulating these acupressure points can help to relieve sinus pain and congestion, and the symptoms of nasal allergy as well. The points shown in Figure F are defined and described below.

1. LI (large intestine) 4—in the webbing between thumb and index finger. To locate the exact point, bring your thumb alongside the index finger; the hump or "meatiest" part of the web is your spot. Stimulate both hands. This point is effective for a problem anywhere in your head, e.g., headache, toothache, eye or vision problem.

2. Extra Bitong—along the edge of the nasal bone in the groove alongside the nose.

3. LI 20—beside the nose at the midpoint of its widest part.

4. ST (stomach) 2—in the tiny notch on the bony ridge below the eye, in line with the pupil.

5. UB (urinary bladder) 2—on the nasal end of the eyebrow in a small notch in the underlying bone.

6. Extra Yin Tang—midway between the nasal ends of the eyebrows.

7. Extra Tai Yang—in the depression of the temple (also a good point to use for headaches).

8. Extra Yu Yao—the middle of the eyebrow, in line with the pupil.

9. Along both sides of the bridge of the nose in the nasal corner of the eye socket. This is not an official Chinese acupressure point, but many sinus patients have obtained relief using it.

The Chinese herbs that are most effective for treating sinuses (they are also used for allergies) are Bi Yan Pian, Pe Min Kan Wan, Seven Forests–Xanthium 12, and Pollen Allergy.

HOMEOPATHIC MEDICINE

Homeopathy is a form of treatment that gently nudges the body toward a healthier state. Its practice was begun in 1820 by Samuel Hahnemann, a German physician, who believed that whatever caused disease would also cure it. The Latin phrase "Similia similibus curantur" (Like shall be cured by like) is the cornerstone of homeopathic medicine. According to Hahnemann, the proper remedy for an illness is that substance which would produce the same set of symptoms in a healthy person that is exhibited in the sick patient. This "Law of Similars" was not original with Hahnemann. The idea had been advanced by philosophers and physicians for thousands of years, and Hahnemann acknowledged his debt to Hippocrates, in whose writings the principle of "like cures like" appears. Hahnemann, however, was the first to build a consistent system of therapeutics based on this principle.

Homeopathy flourished in the 1800s and hasn't changed much since then. The Hahnemann School of Medicine in Philadelphia was originally a school of homeopathic medicine. The advent of rigorous scientific medicine in the United States during this century almost completely eliminated homeopathy. Today, this healing discipline is on the rise all over the world, including this country. The National Center for Homeopathic Medicine in Washington, D.C., estimates that there are roughly 1000 to 2000 practitioners in the United States and that about 300 of them are M.D.s or D.O.s. But homeopathy has fared much better in other parts of the world. One-third of all French physicians practice it. In Britain, members of the royal family have been cared for by homeopathic physicians since the reign of Queen Victoria. Homeopathy is taught and used in hospitals and physicians' offices in Scotland, Germany, Austria, Switzerland, India, Mexico, Chile, Brazil, and Argentina.

Homeopathy uses infinitesimal or micro doses of natural—i.e., mineral, plant, or animal—materials. Some standard homeopathic solutions may be as weak as one part in 100,000. These mixtures have to be vigorously shaken ("succussed") in a carefully prescribed manner in order to be activated. Homeopaths believe that the treatment works, even though such tiny amounts of a substance are used, because even if the substance were reduced to a single molecule, or lost altogether, its "pattern" would remain in the liquid and could produce an effect. Scientific support for this theory was contained in a 1988 issue of the prestigious British journal *Nature*. The publication described a study from a French laboratory headed by a well-known medical research scientist in the fields of allergy and immunology. The research team demonstrated that a solution that had contained a human antibody, yet was so dilute that not a molecule of it was left, had produced a response in human blood cells. Although science cannot explain precisely how this could happen, the reasons why many pharmaceutical drugs, including aspirin, are effective are still largely a mystery as well.

Homeopathic medicines are not required to meet the "safe and effective" standards of the Food and Drug Administration. They are sold by mail, in drugstores, and in health food stores. Most are nonprescription and can legally be advertised as remedies only for self-limiting conditions, such as colds. Prescription homeopathic substances can be dispensed only by someone licensed to prescribe drugs.

Most patients who seek the care of a homeopathic practitioner have a chronic condition that is considered incurable by traditional medicine. An effective homeopathic treatment for both acute and chronic sinusitis is Kali Bichromium 30c every hour for four or five doses. There are others as well. I've recently learned of a homeopathic nasal spray that also works quite well. It's called Euphorbium Nasal Spray, is manufactured in Germany, and is distributed by Biological Homeopathic Industries in Albuquerque, New Mexico.

REFLEXOLOGY

Reflexology is a science that makes use of the fact that there are reflex areas in the feet and hands corresponding to all of the glands, organs, and parts of the body. It employs a unique method of using the thumb and fingers on the reflex areas to relieve stress and tension, improve blood supply and promote the unblocking of nerve impulses, and help the body achieve homeostasis—a state of balance.

Reflexology is a natural, noninvasive therapy that grew out of the theories and techniques of acupuncture and acupressure. From hieroglyphic paintings found on a wall of an ancient Egyptian tomb, there is strong evidence to suggest that reflexology was practiced before 2330 B.C. From other ancient texts, illustrations, and artifacts, it is known that the early Japanese, Indians, and Russians, as well as the Chinese and Egyptians, worked on the feet to promote good health.

But as with Chinese medicine, it was not until the twentieth century that reflexology started to gain acceptance in the Western world. Foot reflexology was introduced in the United States in 1913 by William H. Fitzgerald, M.D., following his discovery of the Chinese method of zone therapy. While serving as the head of the Nose and Throat Department of St. Francis Hospital in Hartford, Connecticut, he developed the modern zone theory of the human body, arguing that some parts of the body correspond to other parts and offering as proof the fact that applying pressure to one area anesthetizes a corresponding area.

In the 1930s, Eunice Ingham, a physiotherapist for Joseph S. Riley, M.D. (a pioneer in the field of zone therapy), used zone therapy in her work with patients. She found the feet to be the most responsive areas for working the zones because they were extremely sensitive. Eventually she "mapped" all the points on the feet that corresponded with points in other parts of the body. She discovered that an alternating pressure applied with the thumb and fingers on the various points on the feet had therapeutic effects far beyond the limited use to which zone therapy had been previously employed, i.e., reduction of pain. Thus reflexology was born.

As with acupuncture, reflexology attempts to strengthen and balance the intangible life energy, *chi* or *qi,* that flows in zones or meridians throughout the body. Reflexologists specify ten energy zones that run the length of the body from head to toe—five on each side of the body ending in each foot and running down the arms into the tips of the fingers. Not only do these zones run lengthwise, but they pass through the body, so

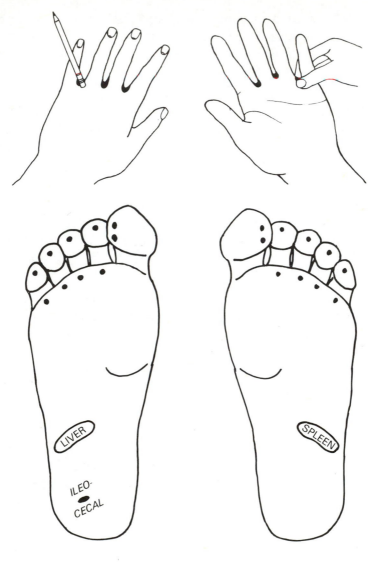

RIGHT FOOT   LEFT FOOT

Figure G. Reflex Points.

that a zone located on the front of the body can also be reached
from behind. All of the organs and parts of the body lie along
one or more of these zones. Stimulating or "working" any
zone in the foot by applying pressure with the thumbs and
fingers affects the entire zone throughout the body. The actual

physical mechanism that controls the ten zones in the body and feet is not fully understood. But it is a fact that reflexology is effective as an adjunct in the treatment of a variety of chronic ailments, probably as a result of its ability to induce deep states of relaxation. With this reduction of stress in the body, there are many potential benefits. Circulation can be improved; toxins and waste products eliminated more easily; energy levels increased; mental alertness, creativity, and productivity heightened.

I can personally attest to the state of relaxation that can result from a reflexology session. I have also known patients suffering from chronic sinusitis who experienced dramatic relief through this treatment modality. Reflex therapy can be administered through alternating finger pressure and/or percussion. This can be applied using the fingers (usually the index finger, with a rotating method of compression massage) and thumb, or using percussion machines. I have a device called a Reflex-Aid (a floor-mounted foot massage machine), equipped with a spiked rubber ball, under my desk. This allows me to passively massage the foot reflexes while I'm working.

For anyone interested in trying this approach as a complement to their holistic health program, I would recommend beginning with a visit to a reflexologist. See how it feels to have your feet worked on by a professional. Figure G illustrates the sinus points on the hands and the feet. Both hands have identical points in the webbing between the fingers. They can be stimulated with the thumb and index finger or even with the eraser of a pencil. Apply the pressure for twenty to thirty seconds and with enough strength to cause some discomfort. The sinus points are the same on the soles of both feet. There are also three other points—liver and ileo-cecal valve (both on the right foot) and spleen (on the left)—that are important in treating the sinuses. Try stimulating all of these points on a daily basis and see what happens. If nothing else, you'll be giving your feet, one of our most abused body parts, some welcome attention.

Chapter 16

Conclusion

Having read this far in the book, you know now that the treatment of sinus disease can encompass the entire spectrum of medicine—from simply taking antibiotics to engaging in a life-transformational process. If you choose, it can involve making the transition from dependence upon the medical profession for your health to the recognition that you are capable of healing yourself. A human being, in fact, is an intrinsically self-healing organism. But we have developed many unhealthy habits that make it much more difficult for us to fully enjoy our lives.

In *Sinus Survival* I have shared with you my approach to health, derived from a healing odyssey that began with my family roots in traditional allopathic medicine and continued through the transition from strict medical science to holism (the transitional stage is osteopathic medicine) to what will become the foundation of the health care system of the future—holistic medicine. What began as a desire to improve the condition of my sinuses has led me to a different style of medical practice; a cure for sinus disease and potentially any other chronic condition; and the recognition of a degree of health I had never imagined possible.

There is nothing really new about this approach, except that medical science is now beginning to explain it and somewhat reluctantly give it its scientific stamp of approval through the field of psychoneuroimmunology. Many so-called primitive cultures, much less technologically developed than our own, have been instinctively practicing variations of holistic medicine for generations. Rather than discard the monumental scientific advances of modern medicine, holistic medicine in the developed world is a comprehensive approach that incorporates everything from ancient healing practices to space-age technologies.

My medical career has involved continual attempts to refine and improve my skills as a physician in order to practice medicine to the best of my ability. As a family doctor, I have spent most of the past twenty years trying to find simple, quick, painless, and effortless remedies to satisfy my patients' requests for fast relief of their discomfort. During the past four years as a holistic physician, however, I've learned that our tremendous desire for the "quick fix" is one of our greatest obstacles to health. The approach I offer in this book synthesizes my family practice orientation as a "fixer" of symptoms, friend, and counselor (time permitting) with the focus of holistic medicine—the physician serving as a facilitator and teacher in the patient's own process of self-healing.

If you are willing to make the commitment to the holistic program, then you will be giving yourself life's greatest gift. Its primary expense seems to be our society's most precious commodity—time. If you're not in a hurry, you've got it made. And you'll probably be surprised to find that the program doesn't take nearly as much time out of your daily schedule as you thought it would. Many of the methods and practices that I have described require only a heightened awareness on your part and no extra time. I'd recommend that you start by choosing only one or possibly two methods in each component of health that require extra time. As you experience the rewards of practicing good health, you will be motivated to choose additional methods and expand your program. The following is an example of what a beginning program could look like with particular respect to the time commitment.

PHYSICAL HEALTH

Eating and drinking are things you already do every day. The recommended diet might entail shopping for food at a different store and spending a bit more time initially on preparing some new dishes. Drinking more water and taking vitamins and herbs requires awareness but negligible extra time. Aerobic exercise at least three times a week for thirty minutes is the major time consumer, but it's worth it. Getting to and from, showering, etc., could make the actual time required for exercise closer to an hour. Averaged over a one-week period, including extra time for food shopping and cooking, physical health would require about **forty minutes** per day.

MENTAL HEALTH

Initially making a list of your goals, desires, and objectives for every realm of holistic health will definitely take some time, but the list serves as your guide for the rest of the program and only has to be done once. After rephrasing the goals into affirmations, reciting or listening to this list twice a day would probably require a total daily time of **five to ten minutes.** Most of the other aspects of mental health—optimism, choice, humor, and forgiveness—entail only greater awareness, much of it derived from the daily recitation of the affirmations.

EMOTIONAL HEALTH

The primary objective of emotional health is to gain a greater awareness of your feelings. You can accomplish this to some extent just by identifying it as one of your goals. Meditation can initially be practiced for five minutes twice a day. An anger-releasing technique—screaming, punching, stamping—can take just a minute or two. These two methods are the ones I would recommend starting with, although participating regularly in a sport or strenuous physical activity could doubly serve to provide aerobic exercise and as a means of playing. The total daily time for emotional health is **ten to fifteen minutes.**

SPIRITUAL HEALTH

To gain a greater sense of God in your daily life, the only extra time initially needed might be to pray and recite psalms. That could take less than **five minutes** a day. Listening to your intuition and gratitude require awareness and slowing down. Lighting candles more often takes no time, and if you meditated, prayed, and recited affirmations while sitting in a hot bath you'd have created the perfect time-efficient holistic health device. Don't forget hugs, another all-purpose healthy quick fix.

SOCIAL HEALTH

The most valuable technique that I'd recommend for feeling more connected to another person is the listening exercise. If you start with doing it once a week for forty minutes, that comes out to less than **six minutes** a day. Having family dinners together requires no extra time but offers an excellent opportunity for relating to your children.

If you can make the commitment to give yourself just over an hour a day to start practicing good health, I can assure you it will make a profound difference in the quality of your life, not to mention how good your sinuses will feel. You will soon develop the understanding that being healthy is much more than merely experiencing the absence of physical disease. As you gain a heightened awareness of each of the components of health, you will learn to be more present with whatever it is you're doing; to experience a greater level of physical fitness; to let go of your ego and old, conditioned behavior patterns; to take risks; to be more childlike and have more fun; to be more accepting of pain; to listen to your intuition and make better choices; to spend more time with supportive people; to be better.able to give to others as well as to receive; to see your life as a mirror reflecting back to you your unconscious thoughts and feelings; to respect and better appreciate your home, the earth, and all of its inhabitants; to trust and have more faith; to have greater control over your life; to live while you're alive! This is a state of being holistically healthy.

References

Adinoff, Allen D. "Difficult Asthma? Look for Sinusitis." *National Jewish Center for Immunology and Respiratory Medicine Medical Scientific Update,* February 1987, pp. 1-5.

Baranowski, Zane. *Free Radicals, Stress, and Antioxidant Enzymes: A Guide to Cellular Health* (pamphlet—no publisher, no date).

Carey, Benedict. "A Jog in the Smog." *Hippocrates,* May/June 1989, pp. 94-96.

Collins, John G. "Prevalence of Selected Chronic Conditions, United States, 1983-1985." *National Center for Health Statistics: Advance Data,* May 24, 1988.

Crowther, Richard L. *Indoor Air: Risks and Remedies.* Denver: Directions Publishing, 1989.

Feltman, John (ed.). *Hands-on Healing: Massage Remedies for Hundreds of Health Problems.* Emmaus, Pennsylvania: Rodale Press, 1989.

Gray, Henry. *Anatomy of the Human Body,* 8th ed. Charles Mayo Goss, ed. Philadelphia: Lea and Febiger, 1967.

Guyton, Arthur C. *Textbook of Medical Physiology.* Philadelphia: W.B. Saunders Company, 1968.

Hay, Louise L. *You Can Heal Your Life.* Santa Monica, California: Hay House, 1984.

Hendeles, Leslie; Weinberger, Miles; and Wong, Lai. "Medical Management of Noninfectious Rhinitis." *American Journal of Hospital Pharmacy,* November 1980, p. 1496.

Hendrix, Harville. *Getting the Love You Want: A Guide for Couples.* New York: Harper and Row, 1988.

Hersch, Patricia. "The Resounding Silence." *The Family Therapy Networker,* July/August 1990, pp. 19-29.

Growald, Eileen Rockefeller, and Allan Luks. "The Healing Power of . . . Doing Good." *American Health,* March 1988, p. 98.

Joy, W. Brugh. *Joy's Way: A Map for the Transformational Journey.* Los Angeles: J.P. Tarcher, 1979.

Kozora, E.J. *American Holistic Medical Association's Nutritional Guidelines.* Seattle, Washington: American Holistic Medical Association, 1987.

Krakovitz, Rob. *High Energy: How to Overcome Fatigue and Maintain Your Peak Vitality.* New York: Ballantine Books, 1986.

Langs, Robert. "Understanding Your Dreams." *New Age Journal,* July/August 1988, pp. 50-83.

National Institute of Allergy and Infectious Diseases. "Sinusitis." Bethesda, Maryland.

Ophir, Dov; Elad, Yigal; Dolev, Zvi; and Geller Bernstein, Carmi. "Effects of Inhaled Humidified Warm Air on Nasal Patency and Nasal Symptoms in Allergy Rhinitis." *Annals of Allergy,* March 1988, pp. 239-242.

Ornstein, Robert, and Sobel, David. *Healthy Pleasures.* New York: Addison-Wesley, 1989.

Patent, Arnold. *You Can Have It All.* Great Neck, New York: Money Mastery, 1984.

Peck, M. Scott. *The Road Less Traveled.* New York: Simon and Schuster, 1978.

Reid, Clyde. *Celebrate the Temporary.* New York: Harper and Row, 1972.

Siegel, Bernie S. *Love, Medicine and Miracles.* New York: Harper and Row, 1986.

South Coast Air Quality Management District. *Where Does It Hurt?: Answers to Questions about Smog and Health.* El Monte, California.

Togias, Alkis G.; Nacierio, Robert M.; Proud, David; Fish, James E.; Adkinson, N. Franklin Jr.; Kagey Sobotka, Anne; Norman, Philip S.; and Lechtenstein, Lawrence M. "Nasal Challenge With Dry Cold Air in Release of Inflammatory Mediators: Possible Mast Cell Involvement." *The American Society for Clinical Investigation,* October 1985, p. 1375.

United States Environmental Protection Agency, Office of Air Quality Planning and Standards Technical Support Division. *National Air Quality and Emissions Trend Report, 1988.* Research Triangle Park, North Carolina, 1990.

Warga, Claire. "You Are What You Think." *Psychology Today,* September 1988, pp. 55-58.

About the Author

Rob Ivker completed his medical training in his hometown at the Philadelphia College of Osteopathic Medicine in 1972. Following a family practice residency at Mercy Medical Center in Denver, he opened a solo practice just outside the "Mile-High City" in 1975. The practice flourished and in 1983 Columbine Medical Center, presently a group of six family physicians, was established. He sold Columbine to Porter Memorial Hospital in 1986 and continued to work for another year as a family doctor and medical director of the center.

Since leaving Columbine and traditional medicine, he has devoted his career to health education and the treatment of chronic disease. The past four years have been spent in training for and practicing holistic medicine, writing—the original and revised editions of *Sinus Survival*, and public speaking.

Dr. Ivker has been twice board-certified by the American Board of Family Practice, is a Fellow of the American Academy of Family Physicians, and is a member of the American Holistic Medical Association.

He lives with his wife, Harriet, and daughters, Julie and Carin, in Littleton, Colorado.

The following products and information are available upon request. Please check the items you'd like, and send a check or money order made payable to "Sinus Survival," along with this order form or a photocopy of it, to Whole Health Press, P.O. Box 620236, Littleton, Colorado, 80162-0236.

____Additional copies of *Sinus Survival*. Cost is $11.95 (includes shipping).

____*Indoor Air: Risks and Remedies*, Richard Crowther. Cost is $19.95 (includes shipping).

The following information is available free of charge:

____Sinus Survival Products (equipment for healthy indoor air), catalog.

____Sinus Survival Spray, brochure.

____Reflex-Aid Foot Massage Machine, brochure.

Please send to:

Name _____

Address _____

City _____ State_____Zip_____